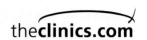

VETERINARY CLINICS

OF NORTH AMERICA

Small Animal Practice

Clinical Pathology and Diagnostic
Techniques

GUEST EDITORS
Robin W. Allison, DVM, PhD
James H. Meinkoth, DVM, PhD

March 2007 • Volume 37 • Number 2

SAUNDERS

An Imprint of Elsevier, Inc.
PHILADELPHIA   LONDON   TORONTO   MONTREAL   SYDNEY   TOKYO

W.B. SAUNDERS COMPANY
A Division of Elsevier Inc.

Elsevier, Inc., 1600 John F. Kennedy Blvd., Suite 1800, Philadelphia, PA 19103-2899

http://www.vetsmall.theclinics.com

VETERINARY CLINICS OF NORTH AMERICA:	**Volume 37, Number 2**
SMALL ANIMAL PRACTICE	**ISSN 0195-5616**
March 2007	**ISBN-13: 978-1-4160-4383-6**
Editor: John Vassallo; j.vassallo@elsevier.com	**ISBN-10: 1-4160-4383-7**

Veterinary Clinics of North America: Small Animal Practice (ISSN 0195-5616) is published bimonthly (For Post Office use only: volume 36 issue 5 of 6) by Elsevier Inc., 360 Park Avenue South, New York, NY 10010-1710. Months of issue are January, March, May, July, September, and November. Business and Editorial offices: 1600 John F. Kennedy Blvd., Suite 1800, Philadelphia, PA 19103-2899. Customer Service Office: 6277 Sea Harbor Drive, Orlando, FL 32887-4800. Periodicals postage paid at New York, NY and additional mailing offices. Subscription prices are $187.00 per year for US individuals, $297.00 per year for US institutions, $94.00 per year for US students and residents, $248.00 per year for Canadian individuals, $373.00 per year for Canadian institutions, $259.00 per year for international individuals, $373.00 per year for international institutions and $127.00 per year for Canadian and foreign students/residents. To receive student/resident rate, orders must be accompanied by name of affiliated institution, date of term, and the *signature* of program/residency coordinator on institution letterhead. Orders will be billed at individual rate until proof of status is received. Foreign air speed delivery is included in all *Clinics* subscription prices. All prices are subject to change without notice. **POSTMASTER**: Send address changes to *Veterinary Clinics of North America: Small Animal Practice*, Elsevier Periodicals Customer Service, 6277 Sea Harbor Drive, Orlando, FL 32887-4800, USA; phone: 1-800-654-2452 [toll free number for US customers], or (+1)(407) 345-4000 [customers outside US]; fax: (+1)(407) 363-1354; email: usjcs@elsevier.com.

Veterinary Clinics of North America: Small Animal Practice is also published in Japanese by Inter Zoo Publishing Co., Ltd., Aoyama Crystal-Bldg 5F, 3-5-12 Kitaaoyama, Minato-ku, Tokyo 107-0061, Japan.

Reprints: For copies of 100 or more, of articles in this publication, please contact the Commercial Reprints Department, Elsevier Inc., 360 Park Avenue South, New York, New York 10010-1710. Tel. (212) 633-3813 Fax: (212) 462-1935, email: reprints@elsevier.com

Veterinary Clinics of North America: Small Animal Practice is covered in *Current Contents/Agriculture, Biology and Environmental Sciences, Science Citation Index, ASCA, Index Medicus, Excerpta Medica,* and *BIOSIS.*

Printed in the United States of America.

ELSEVIER
SAUNDERS

VETERINARY CLINICS
SMALL ANIMAL PRACTICE

Clinical Pathology and Diagnostic Techniques

GUEST EDITORS

ROBIN W. ALLISON, DVM, PhD, Diplomate, American College of Veterinary Pathologists; Assistant Professor of Clinical Pathology, Department of Veterinary Pathobiology, Center for Veterinary Health Sciences, Oklahoma State University, Stillwater, Oklahoma

JAMES H. MEINKOTH, DVM, PhD, Diplomate, American College of Veterinary Pathologists; Professor of Clinical Pathology, Department of Veterinary Pathobiology, Center for Veterinary Health Sciences, Oklahoma State University, Stillwater, Oklahoma

CONTRIBUTORS

ROBIN W. ALLISON, DVM, PhD, Diplomate, American College of Veterinary Pathologists; Assistant Professor of Clinical Pathology, Department of Veterinary Pathobiology, Center for Veterinary Health Sciences, Oklahoma State University, Stillwater, Oklahoma

PAUL R. AVERY, VMD, PhD, Diplomate, American College of Veterinary Pathologists; Assistant Professor, Department of Microbiology, Immunology, and Pathology, College of Veterinary and Biomedical Sciences, Colorado State University, Fort Collins, Colorado

ANNE C. AVERY, VMD, PhD, Assistant Professor and Director, Clinical Immunopathology Service, and Department of Microbiology, Immunology, and Pathology, College of Veterinary and Biomedical Sciences, Colorado State University, Fort Collins, Colorado

GREGORY A. CAMPBELL, MS, DVM, PhD, Diplomate, American College of Veterinary Pathologists; Associate Professor and Chief Pathologist, Oklahoma Animal Disease Diagnostic Laboratory, Oklahoma State University Center for Veterinary Health Sciences, Stillwater, Oklahoma

SHARON A. CENTER, DVM, Diplomate, American College of Veterinary Internal Medcine; Professor, Department of Clinical Sciences, College of Veterinary Medicine, Cornell University, Ithaca, New York

P. CYNDA CRAWFORD, DVM, PhD, Assistant Scientist, Department of Small Animal Clinical Sciences, College of Veterinary Medicine, University of Florida, Gainesville, Florida

SHARON M. DIAL, DVM, PhD, Diplomate, American College of Veterinary Pathologists; Research Scientist, Department of Veterinary Science and Microbiology, Arizona Veterinary Diagnostic Laboratory, University of Arizona, Tucson, Arizona

GREGORY F. GRAUER, DVM, MS, Diplomate, American College of Veterinary Internal Medicine; Professor and Jarvis Chair of Small Animal Internal Medicine, Department of Clinical Sciences, College of Veterinary Medicine, Kansas State University, Manhattan, Kansas

JULIE K. LEVY, DVM, PhD, Diplomate, American College of Veterinary Internal Medicine; Associate Professor, Department of Small Animal Clinical Sciences, College of Veterinary Medicine, University of Florida, Gainesville, Florida

MICHAEL E. MATZ, DVM, MS, Diplomate, American College of Veterinary Internal Medicine; Internist, Veterinary Specialty Clinic of Tucson, Tucson, Arizona

JAMES H. MEINKOTH, DVM, PhD, Diplomate, American College of Veterinary Pathologists; Professor of Clinical Pathology, Department of Veterinary Pathobiology, Center for Veterinary Health Sciences, Oklahoma State University, Stillwater, Oklahoma

LESLIE SAUBER, DVM, Diplomate, American College of Veterinary Dermatology; Veterinary Dermatologist, Tulsa Veterinary Dermatology, Tulsa, Oklahoma

LESLIE C. SHARKEY, DVM, PhD, Diplomate, American College of Veterinary Pathologists; Associate Professor, Department of Veterinary Population Medicine, College of Veterinary Medicine, University of Minnesota, St. Paul, Minnesota

MARY ANNA THRALL, DVM, MS, Diplomate, American College of Veterinary Pathologists; Professor of Veterinary Clinical Pathology, Department of Microbiology, Immunology, and Pathology, College of Veterinary Medicine and Biomedical Sciences, Colorado State University, Fort Collins, Colorado; Professor of Veterinary Clinical Pathology, Department of Pathobiology, Ross University School of Veterinary Medicine, Basseterre, St. Kitts, West Indies

LINDA M. VAP, MT, DVM, Diplomate, American College of Veterinary Pathologists; Instructor and Coordinator, Clinical Pathology Laboratory, Department of Microbiology, Immunology, and Pathology, College of Veterinary Medicine and Biomedical Sciences, Colorado State University, Fort Collins, Colorado

M. GLADE WEISER, DVM, Diplomate, American College of Veterinary Pathologists; Professor, Special Appointment, Department of Microbiology, Immunology, and Pathology, College of Veterinary Medicine and Biomedical Sciences, Colorado State University, Fort Collins; Clinical Pathologist, Heska Corporation, Loveland, Colorado

VETERINARY CLINICS
SMALL ANIMAL PRACTICE

SEVIER
UNDERS

Clinical Pathology and Diagnostic Techniques

CONTENTS   VOLUME 37 • NUMBER 2 • MARCH 2007

Results of many routine laboratory assays supply important diagnostic information and are an important part of patient care in many situations. Ensuring the accuracy of these results is not only important from a diagnostic standpoint but can prevent the frustration inherent when the effort of collecting and submitting samples does not yield interpretable results. This article discusses some of the routinely encountered problems (and how to avoid them) associated with performing the more commonly requested tests: complete blood cell counts, chemistry profiles, coagulation testing, and cytology specimens. The article presents a general discussion of sample collection and handling and then some specific considerations for the handling of the previously mentioned tests.

The typical technologies used in veterinary hematology and biochemical analyzers are reviewed, along with associated advantages and disadvantages. Guidelines for implementing a successful in-clinic laboratory are provided, including criteria for system evaluation and expectations for comparative performance evaluations. The more common problems and limitations associated with in-clinic laboratory diagnostics and how to best prevent them are also discussed.

The design and use of quality control materials and rationale for implementation of a quality monitoring program are discussed. A simplified approach to a quality monitoring program suitable for in-clinic laboratories is presented. Use of blood films and the mean cell hemoglobin concentration value as adjuncts to quality monitoring in hematology is described. Over time, it is hoped that the profession more widely embraces, if not demands, implementation of quality monitoring for in-clinic laboratory diagnostics.

Hematology Without the Numbers: In-Clinic Blood Film Evaluation

Robin W. Allison and James H. Meinkoth

Multimedia components available within this article at www.vetsmall.theclinics.com, March 2007 issue.

Technical advances have made it possible for many private veterinary practices to purchase reasonably priced automated hematology instruments to perform in-clinic blood analyses. Although these instruments can quickly provide "numbers" to the clinician, evaluation of a well-made blood film can often provide information critical to the interpretation of those numbers. Blood film review is essential to identify important abnormalities such as neutrophilic left shifts and toxic change, neoplastic cells, hemoparasites, and erythrocyte morphologic changes that may suggest the cause of an anemia. Additionally, the blood film provides an important quality control measure for the automated hematology results. This article outlines a simple method of blood film evaluation, highlights the most common clinically important abnormalities, and reinforces the importance of blood film evaluation as a quality control measure.

Determining the Significance of Persistent Lymphocytosis

Anne C. Avery and Paul R. Avery

The authors provide a review of current knowledge of lymphocytosis in nonneoplastic conditions. They conclude that the list of major differentials for persistent nonneoplastic lymphocyte expansion in dogs and cats is short and that most of these conditions are relatively uncommon. Persistent lymphocytosis of small, mature, or reactive lymphocytes is most commonly the result of chronic lymphocytic leukemia or lymphoma. The first step in distinguishing nonneoplastic from neoplastic lymphocytosis is immunophenotyping by flow cytometry to determine the phenotypic diversity of the circulating cells. Clonality testing using the polymerase chain reaction for antigen receptor rearrangements assay is a useful second step in cases in which the phenotype data are equivocal. Once the diagnosis of malignancy has been established, the immunophenotype also provides prognostic information in dogs.

Measurement, Interpretation, and Implications of Proteinuria and Albuminuria

Gregory F. Grauer

Proteinuria is a common disorder in dogs and cats that can indicate the presence of chronic kidney disease (CKD) before the onset of azotemia or the presence of more severe CKD after the onset of azotemia. Although a direct pathogenetic link between glomerular disease, proteinuria, and progressive renal damage has not been established, attenuation of proteinuria has been associated with decreased renal functional decline in several studies. There is a need to continue to increase our understanding of the effects of proteinuria on the glomerulus, the tubule, and the interstitium in dogs and cats.

Abnormalities in liver enzymes are commonly encountered in clinical practice. Knowledgeable assessment requires a full understanding of their pathophysiology and provides an important means of detecting the earliest stage of many serious hepatobiliary disorders. The best interpretations are achieved using an integrated approach, combining historical and physical findings with routine and specialized diagnostic procedures and imaging studies. Information in this article provides the foundation, by example, for understanding the reliability of single time point enzyme measurements, the value of sequential measurements, the importance of interpreting the activity of enzymes in light of their half life and tissue of origin, and the influence of the induction phenomenon.

Vaccination of cats against feline immunodeficiency virus (FIV) with a whole-virus vaccine results in rapid and persistent production of antibodies that are indistinguishable from those used for diagnosis of FIV infection. There are no diagnostic tests available for veterinary practitioners at the present time to resolve the diagnostic dilemma posed by use of whole-virus vaccines for protection of cats against FIV. There is a great need for development of commercially available rapid diagnostic tests that conform to differentiation of infected from vaccinated animals standards.

Cytology is a valuable diagnostic tool in veterinary medicine. A review of the literature indicates its utility in evaluation of specific lesions. The information obtained from cytology is greatly enhanced by a good understanding of its advantages and disadvantages and an open and interactive relationship between clinicians and pathologists. Critical selection of appropriate lesions, good sampling technique, quality sample handling, and provision of a complete clinical history and lesion description enhance the utility of the information returned to the clinician by the pathologist. A good cytologic diagnosis is a team effort.

Fungal Diagnostics: Current Techniques and Future Trends

Sharon M. Dial

The diagnosis of fungal disease is a challenge that requires diligent attention to history and clinical signs as well as an astute ability to interpret laboratory data. Because fungal disease can mimic other infectious and neoplastic diseases in clinical presentation, the clinician has to be aware of fungal diseases common locally as well as in other regions of the country. A global approach to the diagnosis of fungal disease that correlates clinical signs as well as physical examination, clinical pathology, and histopathology findings with serology, culture, and the newer immunohistochemical and molecular techniques, where available, is the best approach to optimize the identification of the underlying agent.

Getting the Most from Dermatopathology

Gregory A. Campbell and Leslie Sauber

Dermatohistopathology is one of the most powerful diagnostic tools in clinical dermatology. It is a process in which the veterinary clinician and the veterinary pathologist must consider themselves a team in patient care. The veterinary clinician must know when biopsies are indicated; be able to select lesions to biopsy that are likely to yield diagnostic results; skillfully procure the biopsy samples; and provide the pathologist with an accurate history, clinical description, and clinical differential diagnosis. The pathologist should have particular interest and expertise in dermatohistopathology, be readily accessible to the clinician, and be vigilant in the pursuit of an accurate histologic description and diagnosis.

Index

VETERINARY CLINICS
SMALL ANIMAL PRACTICE

VETERINARY CLINICS
SMALL ANIMAL PRACTICE

Preface

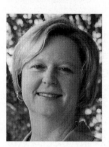
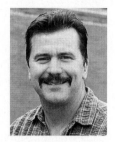

Robin W. Allison, DVM, PhD
James H. Meinkoth, DVM, PhD

Guest Editors

M y passion for clinical pathology was born out of my first career as a veterinary technician, during which I spent 15 years working with talented veterinarians in private practice. Although I enjoyed all aspects of my job, nothing made me happier than to come out of my in-clinic laboratory with hematology, biochemistry, or cytology results that helped to provide a diagnosis and appropriate treatment for one of our patients. Years later, having pursued a DVM degree, residency training and board certification in clinical pathology, as well as a PhD degree and research, I find myself in academia teaching veterinary students and thinking once again about private practice. There are so many diverse diagnostic tests available to private practitioners, and new technology is making it possible to perform more of those tests in the clinic setting. Therefore, I am particularly pleased to coedit, along with my friend and colleague, Dr. Jim Meinkoth, this issue of *Veterinary Clinics of North America: Small Animal Practice* dealing with clinical pathology and diagnostic techniques. We have been able to bring together a remarkable group of pathologists, immunologists, and internists to provide their expertise on a variety of subjects that we hope are of value to veterinarians in private practice. I am especially glad to include articles dealing with in-clinic hematology and clinical chemistry diagnostics, which are becoming increasingly popular as the technology becomes more affordable. In the realm of hematology, my personal fear is that veterinarians have forgotten the value of blood film evaluation instead of relying solely on numbers generated by automated analyzers.

I am indebted to all our contributing authors for their willingness to participate in this project and for their hard work preparing excellent articles, but I must give special thanks to Dr. Mary Anna Thrall. Dr. Thrall was not only

0195-5616/07/$ – see front matter
doi:10.1016/j.cvsm.2006.11.013

a mentor to me during my residency at Colorado State University but was my inspiration to give up my veterinary technician career and return to college and become a veterinary clinical pathologist. As I have told her on more than one occasion, "Mary Anna, this is all your fault!"

Robin W. Allison, DVM, PhD
Department of Veterinary Pathobiology
Center for Veterinary Health Sciences
Oklahoma State University
250 McElroy Hall
Stillwater, OK 74078, USA

E-mail address: robin.allison@okstate.edu

Clinical pathology has fascinated me since I was a veterinary student, when I was taught by Drs. Ron Tyler and Rick Cowell. They shared with me the joy of being able to "solve the puzzle" and started me on this road, for which I remain in their debt. Now, after several years of being at the front of the classroom, I still find what I do as fresh and exciting as ever. I think clinical diagnostics appeals to the Sherlock Holmes in all of us, providing the clues to help us decipher what is happening inside the patient on the examination table.

It is an honor to be a part of the creation of another issue of the *Veterinary Clinics of North America: Small Animal Practice* devoted specifically to diagnostics. I am grateful to all the outstanding authors who contributed their time and expertise in producing excellent articles. I especially want to thank my friend, Dr. Robin Allison, for persuading me to participate in this little adventure. Because I am known to be somewhat "organizationally challenged" and "deadline deficient," I would not have done this alone. She certainly did the lion's share of the planning and oversight of this project and did it extremely well. Finally, I want to thank my wife Tina and son Phillip who put up with me not being able to say "no" to interesting projects that inevitably take some of my time away from them.

James H. Meinkoth, DVM, PhD
Department of Veterinary Pathobiology
Center for Veterinary Health Sciences
Oklahoma State University
250 McElroy Hall
Stillwater, OK 74078, USA

E-mail address: james.meinkoth@okstate.edu

Vet Clin Small Anim 37 (2007) 203–219

VETERINARY CLINICS
SMALL ANIMAL PRACTICE

Sample Collection and Handling: Getting Accurate Results

James H. Meinkoth, DVM, PhD*,
Robin W. Allison, DVM, PhD

Department of Veterinary Pathobiology, Center for Veterinary Health Sciences,
Oklahoma State University, 250 McElroy Hall, Stillwater, OK 74078, USA

Laboratory testing is an integral part of small animal practice; it has become a standard part of wellness examination, preoperative screening, diagnosing disease processes, and assessing the efficacy of treatment or progression of disease. Often, the assumption is made that the results of the various tests being run are accurate and that abnormal results reflect a physiologic change occurring in the patient. Unfortunately, this assumption is not always true. Inaccurate results, from a myriad of causes, are an inherent part of diagnostic testing (although a part that can be minimized). Having inaccurate results is often worse than having no results at all because they can lead to an incorrect diagnosis or result in unnecessary testing and waste of the client's financial resources (or exposure of the patient to unnecessary risks) in the pursuit of the cause of an abnormality that does not exist. Accuracy of test results is extremely important, and limiting the frequency of invalid results is a worthy goal.

Although aberrant test results are sometimes lumped under the heading of "laboratory error," there are many potential sources of error throughout the testing process. This process starts with how the sample is collected, continues with how it is handled until it is run, and finally comes down to the mechanics of how the tests are run (by an outside laboratory or in your clinic). If you are using an outside laboratory to run your samples, it is the laboratory's responsibility to be sure that the methods by which it generates results from your submitted samples are accurate. If you choose to run laboratory tests in your clinic, this becomes your responsibility. People have a great tendency to believe numbers that come out of laboratory instruments (especially expensive instruments); however, unfortunately, they are not always correct. When trying to maintain an in-house laboratory, it takes considerable effort to ensure accurate results. There are two articles in this issue that describe the chemistry and hematology analyzers currently available to the practitioner (article by Weiser

*Corresponding author. E-mail address: james.meinkoth@okstate.edu (J.H. Meinkoth).

0195-5616/07/$ – see front matter
doi:10.1016/j.cvsm.2006.11.008

and colleagues) and the process of quality control to ensure accurate results from these analyzers (article by Weiser and Thrall) should you decide to handle these tests in-clinic. The more experience you have in generating laboratory results, the more likely you are to question them, especially if they do not seem to fit the clinical picture of the patient in front of you (**Box 1**).

Even if you use a professional laboratory, it is still the clinician's responsibility to collect appropriate samples and make sure they are handled properly until received by the laboratory. Often, samples that arrive at the laboratory are not of sufficient quality to generate accurate results. Sometimes, these samples are flagged and not run until the clinician is contacted; many times, however, they are still processed and results are generated. Unfortunately, invalid results cost just as much as valid results, and this can be a great source of frustration. Given the significant expense of many tests, this is an important consideration. A little effort and diligence on the front end can eliminate a lot of frustration and ill will generated when the results obtained cannot be interpreted or do not answer the questions that prompted their collection.

The goal of this article is to discuss some of the routinely encountered problems (and how to avoid them) associated with performing the more commonly requested tests: complete blood cell counts (CBCs), chemistry profiles, coagulation testing, and cytology specimens. The article presents a general discussion of sample collection and handling and then some specific considerations for the handling of the previously mentioned tests.

GENERAL CONCEPTS OF BLOOD SAMPLE COLLECTION AND HANDLING
Sample Collection
Optimally, the patient should be fasted for 12 hours before collecting blood samples to prevent serum lipemia (lipemia is a milky white appearance of serum or plasma caused by increased concentrations of lipids). Transient lipemia is normal after ingestion of a fatty meal, but the magnitude and duration are variable. Fasting lipemia may occur in certain systemic diseases that affect lipid metabolism (eg, diabetes mellitus, pancreatitis, hypothyroidism), and thus may be unavoidable. In these cases, the laboratory may still be able to generate useful results by clearing the lipemia with ultracentrifugation or the addition of materials designed to clear lipemia from the sample (ie, LipoClear; StatSpin, Norwood, Massachusetts) [1]. The use of lipid-clearing products may itself

---

Box 1: General concept

Laboratory tests should always be interpreted in the context of what you already know about the patient (eg, signalment, presenting complaint, physical examination findings). If laboratory results do not fit this scenario, a bit of skepticism is healthy. Repeating the test in question using a new sample is often the wisest first action.

induce artifacts if the analytes being measured bind to lipoproteins and are removed with them [2]. Conversely, postprandial lipemia is best handled by collecting a new specimen. Often, an animal may be brought into the clinic in a nonfasted state because the need to obtain samples for laboratory testing was not anticipated. Many times, the sample is satisfactory depending on the amount and type of food ingested and the time interval that has elapsed. If you plan to run a chemistry profile, it is best to let the sample clot and then centrifuge the sample so that you can inspect the serum to ensure that it is clear and not lipemic (or hemolyzed) before sending it to the laboratory. If the sample is lipemic, the owner can be instructed to fast the animal and return it at a later time, or if the animal is to be hospitalized, another sample can be collected later.

Hemolysis is another common source of artifact. Hemolysis is recognized as a reddish discoloration of serum or plasma resulting from leakage of intracellular constituents from lysed erythrocytes. Sample hemolysis can be the result of a pathologic process in the patient (ie, intravascular hemolytic anemia) but is more commonly the result of in vitro lysis of red blood cells. Hemolysis can induce artifact in a variety of analytes and by different mechanisms. First, hemolysis can increase the serum concentration of any substance that is present in higher concentrations within erythrocytes than in serum. This type of artifact does not depend on the analyzer or methodology used but may vary according to the species and even the breed being tested. A classic example is the effect of hemolysis on serum potassium. Horses have a high concentration of potassium within red blood cells, whereas dogs and cats typically do not. Thus, hemolysis is likely to induce an artifactual hyperkalemia in equine samples but not in canine and feline samples. Some breeds of dogs (eg, Akita, Shiba Inu) have been found to have high intraerythrocytic potassium, however, and thus may show the same artifact as equine samples in response to significant hemolysis. Second, free hemoglobin released by the erythrocytes can interfere with any analyte if the methodology used measures light wavelengths that are also absorbed significantly by hemoglobin. Alternatively, substances released from erythrocytes may interfere with intermediate chemical reactions used to determine the concentration of an analyte. These latter forms of interference are quite variable depending on the analyzer and methodology.

As previously stated, hemolysis is most commonly the result of in vitro lysis that occurs during sample collection, transfer of the sample to the blood tube, or transport of the sample to the laboratory. The good news is that in vitro lysis is potentially avoidable by using larger bore needles to collect samples; avoiding excessive negative pressure during venipuncture; filling blood tubes gently without forcing the sample into the tube; protecting the sample from temperature extremes; and minimizing transport time to the laboratory or, for chemistry profile samples, separating the serum or plasma from the red blood cells before transport to the laboratory.

Because the effects of lipemia and hemolysis often depend on the analyzer and method used, it is difficult to suggest hard and fast guidelines about the effect on particular analytes. Professional laboratories can often supply information concerning the effect of these artifacts on specific tests for their analyzer and methodology. In general, dry chemistry analyzers are much less affected by lipemia than are chemistry analyzers that use liquid reagents. Many in-clinic instruments use dry chemistry reagents (see the article by Weiser and colleagues elsewhere in this issue) and perform well in the face of moderate lipemia or hemolysis. Still, the most reliable way to ensure that a test result has not been artificially affected is to avoid hemolysis or lipemia whenever possible.

The venipuncture should be a clean venipuncture, with a minimum of "fishing around" for the vein. If it is difficult to collect adequate amounts of blood in a reasonable time (common in cats and other animals with small veins), the sample may clot before getting it into the tubes. The presence of small clots in a sample is more of a problem for hematology results (eg, platelet counts) than for chemistry results.

The sample tubes (blood tubes) should be filled adequately. Generally, the degree of vacuum in the tube automatically fills them to the proper level, but it is a good idea to check and make sure the tubes fill consistently. Tubes may not fill properly if the sample has started to clot in the syringe and plugs the needle or if you have previously taken the top off of the tube and released the vacuum. Many tubes have a "fill line" drawn across the label to show you how much blood should be in the tube. Allow the vacuum tubes to fill naturally, or remove the tube stopper and the needle, and gently fill the tube directly from the syringe. Do not force the blood through the needle with excess pressure because this can result in hemolysis. If you remove the stopper from the tube, be sure that it is replaced snugly within the tube. It can also be wise to use a syringe and needle to recreate a vacuum within the tube to avoid the stopper coming off in transit (Fig. 1). If collecting samples for multiple tubes, fill the anticoagulant tubes first and serum (clot) tubes last.

Sample Handling: Blood Collection Tubes

There are a variety of commercially available tubes that can be used to submit samples. The main difference between the various blood collection tubes is whether or not they contain an anticoagulant to prevent the sample from clotting, and if so, which anticoagulant. Most of the tubes are vacuum tubes with a stopper. The color of the stopper generally indicates the type of anticoagulant added and is fairly consistent from manufacturer to manufacturer, although there is some variation. The following section discusses the commonly used blood tubes and some factors to consider when using them.

Clot tubes (serum tubes, "red-top" tubes)

When blood is put into a serum tube, you can submit it to the laboratory "as is" or you can centrifuge it, collecting the serum and transferring it to another tube for transport to the laboratory. Separating the serum is recommended if transport to is going to be prolonged (overnight or longer) to prevent artifactual changes in certain analytes and, more importantly, to prevent hemolysis

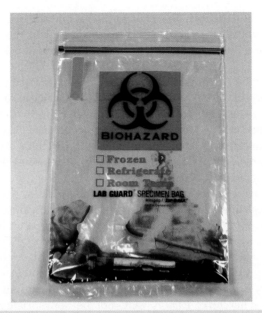

Fig. 1. Sample submitted for a CBC. The stopper was removed to fill the tube and not adequately replaced before mailing.

of the sample. This is discussed further in the section on chemistry profiles. To collect the serum, it is important to let the blood sit for 15 to 20 minutes (preferably at 37°C in a heat block or heated water bath) before centrifugation. This allows time for the clot to form and retract well. If the sample is centrifuged before adequate clot retraction, a fibrin clot may form in the serum, resulting in a gel rather than liquid serum. At this point, it is difficult to recover sufficient quantities of serum, and you often have to collect a new sample. Some red-top tubes contain a "clot activator" to accelerate the coagulation process and reduce the time required to process the sample.

Serum is the standard sample submitted for chemistry profiles, although it can also be used for serologic titers, serum protein electrophoresis, and some endocrine tests among others. Red-top tubes are sometimes used to submit samples for culture. In such instances, it is important to note that some red-top tubes have sterile interiors, although others do not.

Ethylenediaminetetraacetic acid tubes ("purple-top" tubes)
Ethylenediaminetetraacetic acid (EDTA) is an anticoagulant that acts by binding calcium (and other divalent cations), which is required by many of the enzymatic reactions in the coagulation cascade. Most anticoagulants, except for heparin, work in this manner.

EDTA is the anticoagulant of choice for most routine hematology. In addition to its anticoagulant effects, EDTA helps to preserve cell morphology (ideal for blood films) and inhibits bacterial proliferation. Because of this, EDTA should be used whenever cytologic analysis of a sample is desired. In addition to CBCs, common instances include evaluation of pleural, pericardial, or peritoneal effusions.

Plasma from EDTA samples can be used to measure select serum chemistries as well, such as blood urea nitrogen (BUN), glucose and total protein. Although serum or heparinized samples are preferred for performing complete chemistry profiles, many basic "quick assessment tests" can be run from EDTA plasma in patients from whom collection of larger volumes of blood is difficult (eg, small cats). This may be sufficient for presurgical screening in a young clinically healthy patient.

Obviously, plasma from EDTA-anticoagulated samples cannot be used to measure serum calcium (Ca^{++}) concentration. Also, potassium (K^+) concentration cannot be accurately measured because the EDTA in anticoagulant tubes is typically in the form of a potassium salt (K_2-EDTA or K_3-EDTA). Potassium concentration is markedly increased if an EDTA sample is tested (ie, often >20 mEq/L) [3]. EDTA may also interfere with the assay of some enzyme activities, producing falsely decreased results for alkaline phosphatase, lipase, and creatine kinase [3]. Therefore, EDTA may not be appropriate for these tests. Unlike Ca^{++} and K^+, however, the effects on enzyme assays seem to depend on the analyzer and methodology used [3].

Heparin tubes ("green-top" tubes)
Heparin is another anticoagulant and is the only commonly used anticoagulant that does not work by chelating calcium. Heparin potentiates the activity of antithrombin, a natural anticoagulant found in the blood. Antithrombin binds to and inactivates not only thrombin (factor II) but most of the other enzymatic coagulation factors as well. Because heparin does not chelate calcium, it does not interfere with the assay of calcium or the enzymes that require divalent cations. Heparinized plasma can thus be used to run a full chemistry profile. Although serum and heparinized plasma yield similar results on most analytes on a routine biochemical profile, some differences have been noted, including increases in albumin and decreases in potassium and ionized calcium [3].

The main advantage of using heparinized plasma rather than serum is that the blood collected into a red-top tube must sit for approximately 20 minutes to ensure clot formation. Heparinized plasma can be centrifuged immediately and the plasma removed, allowing for more rapid processing. Several heparin salts (eg, sodium heparin, lithium heparin) are used in commercially available blood tubes. Lithium heparin is the preferred type of heparin for most uses because it does not alter the concentration of routinely evaluated electrolytes.

Although EDTA is typically used for CBCs because it does a better job preserving cell morphology, EDTA causes hemolysis in blood samples from some species of birds and reptiles. In these cases, blood samples for CBCs are collected in heparin.

Citrate tubes ("blue-top" tubes)

Citrate is another commonly used anticoagulant, which also acts by binding calcium. Citrate is used to collect samples for routine coagulation tests that are based on measuring the time to clot formation because its anticoagulant effects are easily reversible on addition of calcium to the sample [4]. These tests include the prothrombin time (PT), partial thromboplastin time (PTT), thrombin time (TT), and quantitative fibrinogen determination. Citrated plasma can also be used in assays for concentrations of D-dimers, specific coagulation factors (ie, factor VIII concentration), or von Willebrand factor. When collecting blood for any coagulation test, it is important to have a clean venipuncture so that the sample is not contaminated with tissue factor from tissues surrounding the vein. Contamination of samples with tissue factor can initiate coagulation and shorten coagulation times.

Compared with the other tubes, there is a relatively large volume of anticoagulant in the citrate tubes. It is thus critical that these tubes be filled to the proper level. There should be a 9:1 ratio of blood to citrate. If these tubes are underfilled, there is a relative excess of anticoagulant in the sample, which could potentially prolong the PT and PTT results.

A similar phenomenon occurs in animals with polycythemia (erythrocytosis). If a patient has a markedly increased hematocrit, there is less plasma for a given volume of whole blood. Less plasma volume again results in a relative excess of anticoagulant. Mild prolongations in PT and PTT are observed in animals with an increased hematocrit.

Activated clotting or coagulation time tubes ("gray-top" tubes)

ACT stands for activated clotting time or activated coagulation time, a relatively simple test of coagulation. ACT tubes contain diatomaceous earth, which activates the intrinsic coagulation cascade. By putting blood in an ACT tube and timing how long it takes to clot, you are assessing the factors in the intrinsic and common coagulation pathways. The ACT tube tests essentially the same factors as the PTT, but it can be run in-clinic without the need for specialized instruments.

As with any coagulation test, it is important to have a clean venipuncture. The manufacturer recommends a two-tube method using a vacuum tube system in which the first 2 mL of blood is collected in one tube, which is discarded; a second tube is then filled with 2 mL of blood for ACT evaluation. The purpose of discarding the first 2 mL of blood is to eliminate any blood that has been contaminated with tissue factor during venipuncture. One study in cats found no difference in ACT using a one-tube system (in which the first sample of blood is evaluated) versus a two-tube system [5]. A one-tube system is technically easier to perform, especially in uncooperative or small patients.

Because the ACT tube initiates the intrinsic coagulation pathway, this test must be performed immediately on collection of the blood sample. The tube should be kept at 37°C, ideally by putting it in a heat block or water bath, although simply holding the tube in the axilla of the operator is an alternative.

After an initial incubation of 45 to 60 seconds, the tube is inverted every 10 seconds and checked for clot formation. Normal dogs clot in less than approximately 120 seconds [6]. Normal cats clot in less than approximately 165 seconds [5].

Sodium fluoride tubes ("gray-top" tubes)
These tubes contain sodium fluoride (NaF) and potassium oxalate (Ox). Ox is an anticoagulant that works by chelating calcium. NaF is a chemical that inhibits many of the enzymes involved in glycolysis, which stops metabolism of glucose by cells in the blood sample. Blood samples collected in NaF tubes are used to get an accurate measurement of blood glucose without the need to separate serum or plasma from cells. In addition to inhibiting the use of glucose, NaF inhibits the production of lactate. NaF/Ox tubes are therefore also used when determination of serum lactate concentration is desired. Blood collected in a fluoride tube maintains a stable glucose concentration for at least 24 hours at room temperature and 48 hours in the refrigerator [4]. Lactate was shown to be stable at room temperature in feline samples for at least 8 hours [7]. Fluoride tubes are most useful when performing a glucose response curve in a diabetic patient. Multiple samples can be collected over a period of hours and then sent to the laboratory for glucose determinations in a single batch.

It is important to note that although glucose concentrations remain stable in NaF tubes, glucose concentrations measured in fluoride tubes are artificially lower than concentrations measured from serum in many species [7]. Collection of blood in fluoride tubes results in red blood cell shrinkage and lysis. The shift of intraerythrocytic fluid to plasma results in a decrease in hematocrit and subsequent dilution of some serum analytes, including glucose. In a study of cats, glucose concentrations measured from NaF/Ox plasma were approximately 12% lower than those from paired serum samples in normoglycemic animals [7]. The magnitude of this difference was greater in hyperglycemic animals, averaging 14% lower in a group of diabetic cats [7]. This difference needs to be considered when using NaF/Ox tubes. Certainly, glucose concentrations in samples collected at various times from the same patient should not be used for comparison if different sample types were used for the glucose assay.

Sample Handling: Submission
It is important to be sure that the specimen tube is clearly labeled. Generally, the owner's last name, patient name, and clinic or clinician's name should be included. The date on which the sample was collected should also be included on the tube or on the submittal form in case there is a delay in delivery to the laboratory. Often, samples are received by the laboratory labeled only with the patient's name or even totally unlabeled, which increases the possibility for confusion and misreported results. If anticoagulated plasma is removed from red blood cells and transferred to a serum tube, the type of anticoagulant used should be noted to avoid anticoagulant-induced artifacts in serum chemistries.

Whenever a serum or plasma sample is mailed to an outside laboratory, it is preferable to centrifuge the sample and remove the serum or plasma and place

it in a separate clean tube to prevent artifactual changes. For some tests, samples need to be frozen or sent with an ice pack. It is best to check with the laboratory regarding specific requirements when requesting an assay that you do not routinely run.

Making good-quality blood films to send along with your CBC is highly desirable. Some changes occur in the cells over time, even when collected in EDTA. Making fresh air-dried blood films prevents these artifacts from occurring. This is discussed further in the section on CBCs (see the article by Allison and Meinkoth elsewhere in this issue). If there is going to be a significant delay between collection and submission to the laboratory, the EDTA tube should be refrigerated (but never frozen). Blood films must not be refrigerated. The quality of unfixed air-dried smears does not change significantly for several days to weeks.

If samples are sent through a mailing service, adequate packaging is needed to ensure that the samples arrive at the laboratory unbroken. Glass slides should be placed in rigid plastic (Fig. 2) or polystyrene foam (Fig. 3) containers. The common flat cardboard slide holders (Fig. 4) do not adequately protect the slides, and the slides often arrive at the laboratory broken unless they are subsequently packaged in a sturdy outside container. Similarly, blood tubes should be packaged in a sturdy container, such as a cardboard box or a polystyrene foam mailer.

Most mailing services have specific packaging requirements for handling biologic specimens, including animal blood. Typically, the packaging must consist of a leak-proof primary receptacle (often the blood tube), leak-proof secondary packaging, and sturdy outer packaging. In addition, liquid samples must be surrounded by sufficient absorbent material to absorb the entire contents should any leak or release of liquid occur. Most overnight courier services have dedicated clear plastic "clinical specimen" or "biologic specimen"

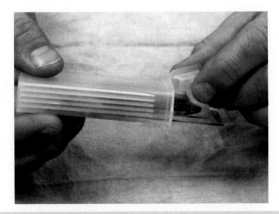

Fig. 2. Rigid plastic slide mailers can hold five to six slides and provide adequate protection during mailing.

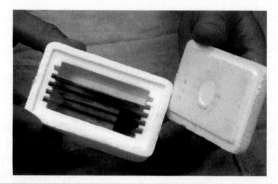

Fig. 3. Polystyrene foam mailers provide adequate protection for slides or tubes during mailing and can hold up to 10 slides (2 slides can fit in each slot). These containers are also large enough to hold small EDTA or serum tubes containing liquid sample.

envelopes that must be used rather than the standard envelopes used for printed material. It is best to contact the courier for specific requirements.

SAMPLE COLLECTION AND HANDLING FOR SPECIFIC TESTS
Complete Blood Cell Counts
Clots and platelet clumps
As mentioned previously, avoidance of clots and platelet clumping is extremely important for accurate CBC results. Platelet clumps and microclots can significantly alter results of the CBC. The most common artifact is a spuriously decreased platelet count (which can be markedly reduced). Whenever a low platelet count is present (especially in cats), the quantitative platelet count from the automated analyzer should be compared with a subjective estimate of platelet numbers from a well-made blood film, including an assessment for

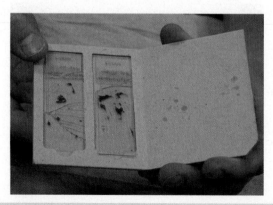

Fig. 4. Thin cardboard slide holders do not provide adequate protection during mailing. Slides are often received broken.

the presence of platelet clumps (this procedure is detailed in the article by Allison and Meinkoth elsewhere in this issue). Microclots within the sample can lead to an erroneously decreased red blood cell count, which reduces the hematocrit (hematocrit is calculated from the red blood cell count and mean cell volume by most automated analyzers). Larger clots invalidate the leukocyte count or, worse, block the hematology analyzer tubing. If you perform in-clinic CBCs on an automated analyzer, always carefully check the sample by gently rocking the tube back and forth while observing for clots before running the sample through the instrument.

To avoid these problems, the CBC sample should be collected from a clean venipuncture, the sample should be collected in a minimal amount of time, the EDTA tube should be filled first if blood has been collected for multiple tubes by means of a syringe rather than directly into vacuum tubes, and the sample must be thoroughly but gently mixed with the anticoagulant immediately after filling the tube. A clean venipuncture is easy to recommend but may be difficult or impossible to achieve in small or uncooperative patients. Furthermore, significant platelet clumping may occur in feline samples even with the best of collections. In one report, 71% of feline CBCs performed using an impedance counter during a 1-year period had decreased automated platelet counts, whereas only 3.1% of these animals were thought to be truly thrombocytopenic based on estimation of platelet counts from blood films [8]. Given this high rate of artifact, estimation of the platelet count from the blood film is an important quality control measure for feline samples (see the article by Allison and Meinkoth elsewhere in this issue). If blood is being collected for hematology and clinical chemistry but the process of obtaining sufficient blood is taking longer than expected, it is often beneficial to terminate the venipuncture when enough blood for just the CBC has been obtained. The EDTA tube can be filled, and a sample for clinical chemistries can be collected from a separate venipuncture. Finally, adequate mixing of the blood and anticoagulant is important. EDTA tubes may contain liquid EDTA or powdered EDTA sprayed onto the entire inner surface of the tube. The sample must be mixed several times by inversion, or if smaller quantities have been obtained, the tube should be rolled so that the sample saturates the entire inner surface of the tube. This should be done in a gentle manner; the tube should never be shaken.

Underfilling tubes

Inadequate filling of EDTA tubes is a common problem, especially when collecting samples from cats and smaller dogs. Commercially available tubes may range from a capacity of less than 1 mL to 10 mL. Significantly underfilling a tube can cause marked artifactual changes in several parameters. With liquid EDTA tubes, there is some degree of dilution artifact. In addition, EDTA is hypertonic and causes water to leave red blood cells, resulting in shrinkage of the cells. This can result in a significant reduction in the apparent packed cell volume (PCV) if the tube is filled with only a fraction of the required amount. Cell shrinkage caused by underfilling a tube may result in decreases in PCV or hematocrit concentrations and mean corpuscular volume (MCV), along with an increase in mean corpuscular hemoglobin concentration (MCHC). Most laboratories require that the EDTA tubes be filled to at least 50% of the intended volume. Microcontainers that are designed to hold as little as 0.25 mL (250 μL) of whole blood are available. These are recommended if the sample size is limited to avoid the previously mentioned artifacts. Table 1 demonstrates the effect of various degrees of underfilling an EDTA tube with blood from a normal dog. The effects may be more pronounced in an anemic animal.

Aging artifact

If hematology samples are run within 1 to 2 hours of collection, artifact from delayed sample processing is generally not a problem. If samples are being sent by overnight courier or, worse, by regular mail, however, significant changes can occur during the transit time. If samples are not going to be processed within approximately 1 hour, blood films should be prepared and the remainder of the sample should be refrigerated. Air-dried unfixed blood films should be sent unstained to the laboratory, providing a sample with good cell morphology even if processing is delayed. Blood films should not be refrigerated. If they are placed in a refrigerator, condensation may occur on the slides and result in lysis of the cells.

Artifacts associated with delayed processing are especially pronounced in the qualitative assessment of the blood smear. Leukocytes undergo aging artifact that, when mild, can make evaluation of toxic changes and left shifts difficult and, when marked, can make identification of the various leukocytes impossible. The rate at which cells undergo degeneration is quite variable and seems to depend on the type of cells present as well as ambient temperature. Immature

Table 1
Effect of underfilling a liquid K_3–ethylenediaminetetraacetic acid tube on selected erythrocyte parameters[a]

Parameter	Sample volume (in 4-mL tube)			Change (in 0.5-mL sample)
	4 mL	1 mL	0.5 mL	
Hct (%)	56.3	52.8	51.9	7.8%
RBCs ($\times 10^6$ cells/μL)	7.61	7.30	7.36	3.2%
Hgb (g/dL)	18.3	17.8	17.7	3.2%
MCV (fL)	74	72.3	70.5	4.7%
MCHC (g/dL)	32.5	33.7	34.2	5.2%

Abbreviations: Hct, hematocrit; Hgb, hemoglobin; MCHC, mean corpuscular hemoglobin concentration; MCV, mean corpuscular volume; RBCs, red blood cells.

[a]Blood sample was from a clinically normal blood donor dog, and the analysis was performed on a Cell-Dyn 3500 (Abbott Laboratories, Abbott Park, Illinois) automated hematology analyzer. Note that the calculated hct concentration is relatively more affected than the RBC count or Hgb concentration because the hct concentration is affected by sample dilution in the EDTA and shrinkage of the RBCs because of hypertonicity of the EDTA solution, whereas the RBC count and Hgb concentration are affected only by sample dilution.

blast cells from an animal with hematopoietic neoplasia can undergo significant degeneration in as little as 24 hours. Fig. 5 demonstrates this effect in an animal with stage V lymphoma. This animal had a total nucleated cell count of 74,000 cells/μL. In films made immediately after collection, numerous large, blastic, lymphoid cells were easily seen in every field. In films made when the EDTA blood sample was received (less than 24 hours later), neutrophils and many degenerated cells were present but neoplastic cells were no longer evident.

Another notable artifact that occurs with storage of blood is that certain hemoparasites dissociate from the red blood cells. Fig. 6 shows blood films made immediately and 24 hours after collection of blood from a cat with *Mycoplasma haemofelis* (*Hemobartonella felis*) infection. In the films made immediately after collection, the typical chains and ring forms of basophilic parasites can be seen associated with many of the red blood cells. In the films made when the EDTA blood sample was received at the laboratory, the parasites have not only "fallen off" the erythrocytes but have changed in appearance as well. This can make confident identification of these organisms difficult. Although many other morphologic changes can occur, these examples demonstrate the benefit of preparing blood films at the time of sample collection. Refrigeration of the EDTA blood sample slows but does not prevent these changes.

In addition to morphologic changes, quantitative changes may occur over time. Platelets can aggregate, leading to a falsely decreased platelet count. Also, erythrocytes may swell significantly, increasing the MCV and hematocrit and decreasing the MCHC within 24 hours [9,10]. Changes in leukocytes are more variable, but aged leukocytes eventually lyse, resulting in decreased leukocyte counts.

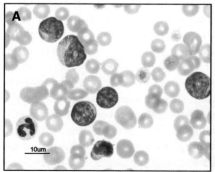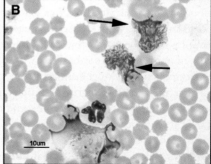

Fig. 5. Blood films from a dog with stage V lymphoma (white blood cell count = 74,000 cells/μL) demonstrate the importance of mailing premade slides along with CBC samples (or fluid cytology samples). (A) Slide made by the clinician at the time the sample was collected. Most of the leukocytes are large immature lymphoid cells. (B) Slide made when the same sample arrived at the laboratory by means of overnight courier (<24 hours later). Neutrophils are recognizable, but the neoplastic cells appear only as bare nuclei of ruptured cells (*arrows*).

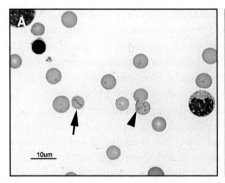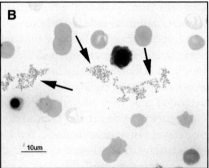

Fig. 6. Blood films from a cat with *Mycoplasma haemofelis* infection show the artifact associated with sample storage time on some hemoparasites. (A) Blood films made immediately
after sample collection show numerous parasites, including ring forms (*arrowhead*) and chains
(*arrow*) associated with the erythrocytes. (B) Blood film made from the same sample when received by the laboratory less than 24 hours after collection. No parasites are evident on erythrocytes. Extracellular organisms are seen as aggregates of pink granular material (*arrows*).

Chemistry Profiles

If the serum is not separated from the cells of the clot, artifactual changes occur
over time. One of the most consistent artifacts is that the glucose concentration
decreases because of use of glucose by the erythrocytes and leukocytes for energy. Glucose concentration decreases by approximately 10% per hour at room
temperature if serum is left in contact with blood cells [4]. Serum Pi (inorganic
phosphate, phosphorous) can increase over time as cells metabolize ATP to
ADP and Pi, with the formed Pi being released into the serum. Other changes
can also occur but are more variable.

A more significant problem associated with leaving serum in contact with
blood cells is that erythrocytes lyse, resulting in hemolysis of the sample. Because most assays are based on absorbance of light transmitted through the
sample, hemolysis can markedly interfere with many tests, depending on the
type of analyzer and methodology used. Hemolysis almost always occurs in un-
separated samples over sufficient time but happens more quickly when the ambient temperature is high (ie, samples mailed in the summer). Hemolysis also
seems to occur more quickly in some animals that are severely ill. In general,
it is best to separate the serum yourself and transfer it to another red-top tube if
the sample has to be mailed to the laboratory. This not only helps to prevent
hemolysis associated with transit but allows you to evaluate the sample for lipemia and preexisting hemolysis from sample collection.

If serum is separated from red blood cells and refrigerated, most analytes on
a routine chemistry profile are stable for 24 to 48 hours.

Coagulation Testing

Two main considerations regarding sample handling for coagulation testing are
adequate filling of the tube and, again, timely processing of the samples. As

previously discussed, citrate tubes have a relatively large volume of anticoagulant. It is important that citrate tubes be filled to their intended volume to prevent artifactual prolongation of the test results.

Coagulation factors are also labile and degrade in vitro over time. It is commonly recommended that citrated plasma used for coagulation testing be kept cool, separated from red blood cells, and assayed within 30 minutes to 4 hours of collection [11–13]. If performing the assays in this amount of time is not feasible, the separated plasma can be frozen (never freeze whole blood) and sent to the laboratory on a cold pack.

Although these recommendations make intuitive sense and are probably safest to ensure sample quality of all specimens, several studies of human and canine samples suggest that most samples for PT and PTT may be stable for much longer periods [14–17]. Studies on canine samples suggest that valid PT and PTT results can be obtained from citrated plasma (removed from red blood cells) stored for up to 48 hours when refrigerated [14] or even at room temperature [15].

Cytology Samples

A complete discussion of collecting and submitting cytology samples is beyond the scope of this article. Other more detailed discussions are available in a previous issue of *Veterinary Clinics of North America: Small Animal Practice* [18]. A few points are worthy of discussion, however.

Air-dried slides for routine cytologic evaluation made from fine-needle aspirates or impression smears are relatively stable for several days without any special handling. Slides should not be fixed with heat or alcohol before submission to the laboratory. The main consideration concerning sample handling is protecting the slides during transport, as previously discussed. Additionally, it is important that unstained slides (of any type) be protected from formalin fumes, which can prevent adequate staining and make evaluation of the sample impossible. For this reason, unstained slides should never be shipped in the same package as a formalin-fixed sample, even when in supposedly "airtight" containers.

Fluid samples for cytology (peritoneal, pleural, and pericardial) are more prone to artifact than are slides made from solid tissue lesions. All fluids intended for cytologic analysis should be submitted in EDTA and refrigerated until sent. Many fluid samples submitted in serum tubes are uninterpretable. Evaluation of fluid samples typically involves determining the nucleated cell count, protein concentration, and cytologic analysis. If the lesion is inflammatory, fluids placed in serum tubes may clot, invalidating cells counts. Also, with no preservative, significant morphologic changes can occur in as little as 24 hours (depending on such factors as the type of cells present and the ambient temperature). Even if the cells are not overtly lysed, evaluation of cells for neoplastic criteria can be hindered by aging artifacts that occur in the cells present. Finally, EDTA can help to prevent overgrowth of bacteria (pathogens or contaminants) during transport. If a bacterial culture is desired, a portion of the sample should be retained and placed in a sterile tube or transport medium in addition to the portion for cytology placed in an EDTA tube.

Even when samples are placed in EDTA, cells undergo degeneration over time. As with blood samples, making smears from the fluid at the time of collection is the best way to preserve cell morphology. Unlike whole blood, however, the cellularity of cytology samples can be extremely variable, and this affects how slides should be made. Samples that are turbid or cloudy are probably of high cellularity. In this instance, making direct smears (similar to making blood films) is generally adequate, because cell density should be sufficient for evaluation. If the sample is relatively clear, however, the cellularity of the sample is probably low and some method of concentrating the cells is important. If sufficient fluid has been obtained, concentrated preparations can be made by centrifuging a portion of the sample in a low-speed centrifuge, decanting most of the supernatant, resuspending the sediment, and then making direct smears from the resulting suspension (similar to preparing a urine sediment). It is still important to make one or two direct smears from which the cellularity of the sample can be estimated. Cell counts generated on automated hematology analyzers from body cavity effusion samples are sometimes erroneous because of the physical properties of the sample, and it is always important to compare automated cell counts with an assessment of cellularity from a direct smear. The direct and concentrated smears should be submitted to the laboratory unstained, along with the fluid in EDTA.

SUMMARY

Results of many routine laboratory assays supply important diagnostic information and are an important part of patient care in many situations. Ensuring the accuracy of these results is not only important from a diagnostic standpoint but can prevent the frustration inherent when the effort of collecting and submitting samples does not yield interpretable results. Fortunately, many of the most common sources of artifacts are easily avoidable. The most important considerations discussed are selection of appropriate tubes in which to submit the sample, minimizing transport time, and taking appropriate steps (eg, refrigeration, preparation of premade smears, adequate packaging) to minimize artifacts when prolonged transport time is unavoidable. Finally, evaluation of sample quality (eg, checking for clots in EDTA samples, evaluating serum for hemolysis or lipemia) can allow for collection of additional samples while the patient is still available.

References

[1] Thomas JS. Introduction to serum chemistries: artifacts in biochemical determinations. In: Willard MD, Tvedten H, editors. Small animal clinical diagnosis by laboratory methods. 4th edition. Philadelphia: WB Saunders; 1999. p. 113–6.
[2] Meyer DJ, Harvey JW. Clinical chemistry. In: Meyer DJ, Harvey JW, editors. Veterinary laboratory medicine: interpretation and diagnosis. 3rd edition. Philadelphia: WB Saunders; 2004. p. 145–55.
[3] Ceron JJ, Martinez-Subiela S, Hennemann C, et al. The effects of different anticoagulants on routine canine plasma biochemistry. Vet J 2004;167(3):294–301.

[4] Young DS, Bermes EW Jr. Specimen collection and other preanalytical variables. In: Burtis CA, Ashwood ER, editors. Tietz fundamentals of clinical chemistry. 5th edition. Philadelphia: WB Saunders; 2001. p. 30–54.

[5] Bay JD, Scott MA, Hans JE. Reference values for activated coagulation time in cats. Am J Vet Res 2000;61(7):750–3.

[6] Byars TD, Ling GV, Ferris NA, et al. Activated coagulation time (ACT) of whole blood in normal dogs. Am J Vet Res 1976;37(11):1359–61.

[7] Christopher M, O'Neill S. Effect of specimen collection and storage on blood glucose and lactate concentrations in healthy, hyperthyroid and diabetic cats. Vet Clin Pathol 2000; 29(1):22–8.

[8] Norman EJ, Barron RCJ, Nash AS, et al. Prevalence of low automated platelet counts in cats: comparison with prevalence of thrombocytopenia based on blood smear estimation. Vet Clin Pathol 2001;30(3):137–40.

[9] Furtanello T, Tasca S, Caldin M, et al. Artifactual changes in canine blood following storage, detected using the ADVIA 120 hematology analyzer. Vet Clin Pathol 2006;35(1):42–6.

[10] Medailli C, Briend-Marchal A, Braun JP. Stability of selected hematology variables in canine blood kept at room temperature in EDTA for 24 and 48 hours. Vet Clin Pathol 2006;35(1): 18–23.

[11] Stockham SL, Scott MA. Hemostasis. In: Stockham SL, Scott MA, editors. Fundamentals of veterinary clinical pathology. Ames (IA): Iowa State Press; 2002. p. 155–225.

[12] Meyer DJ, Harvey JW. Evaluation of hemostasis: coagulation and platelet disorders. In: Meyer DJ, Harvey JW, editors. Veterinary laboratory medicine: interpretation and diagnosis. 3rd edition. Philadelphia: WB Saunders; 2004. p. 107–31.

[13] Topper MJ, Welles EG. Hemostasis. In: Latimer KS, Mahaffey EA, Prasse KW, editors. Duncan and Prasse's veterinary laboratory medicine. 4th edition. Ames (IA): Iowa State Press; 2003. p. 99–135.

[14] Smalko D, Johnstone IB, Crane S. Submitting canine blood for prothrombin time and partial thromboplastin time determinations. Can Vet J 1985;26:135–7.

[15] Furlanello T, Caldin M, Stocco A, et al. Stability of stored canine plasma for hemostasis testing. Vet Clin Pathol 2006;35(2):204–7.

[16] Rao LV, Okorodudu AO, Petersen JR, et al. Stability of prothrombin time and activated partial thromboplastin time tests under different storage conditions. Clin Chim Acta 2000;300: 13–21.

[17] Adcock D, Kressin D, Marlar RA. The effect of time and temperature variables on routine coagulation tests. Blood Coagul Fibrinolysis 1998;9(6):463–70.

[18] Meinkoth JH, Cowell RL. Sample collection and preparation in cytology: increasing diagnostic yield. Vet Clin North Am Small Anim Pract 2002;32(6):1187–207.

Perspectives and Advances in In-Clinic Laboratory Diagnostic Capabilities: Hematology and Clinical Chemistry

M. Glade Weiser, DVM[a,b,*], Linda M. Vap, MT, DVM[a],
Mary Anna Thrall, DVM, MS[a,c]

[a]Department of Microbiology, Immunology, and Pathology, College of Veterinary Medicine and Biomedical Sciences, Colorado State University, Fort Collins, CO 80523, USA
[b]Heska Corporation, 3760 Rocky Mountain Avenue, Loveland, CO 80538, USA
[c]Department of Pathobiology, Ross University School of Veterinary Medicine, Basseterre, St. Kitts, West Indies

TECHNOLOGIC EVOLUTION AND TRENDS

Evolution of laboratory diagnostic instrumentation is driven predominantly by human health care diagnostic market needs. Large central diagnostic laboratory instrumentation systems have evolved to become more automated, capable of higher throughput, and highly sophisticated in test menus and information management capability. The managed health care system in the United States drives most diagnostic testing to large centralized facilities. In contrast, the instrumentation market for small laboratories and physician offices outside North America has driven the development of much smaller systems to meet those needs. These small systems have simultaneously found their way into the "point of care" veterinary market. Over the past 20 years, dramatic progress in reduction of the size, complexity, and cost of laboratory instrumentation for hematology and clinical chemistry has made migration of this technology to small facilities progressively more feasible. This has been made possible by the advances in microprocessor control, miniaturization of fluidics, and microfabrication of mechanical devices. Likewise, improvement in signal measurement and processing has improved precision, accuracy, and general reliability in many systems. This progressive trend has resulted in the ability to move relatively sophisticated diagnostic capability from the central laboratory to the veterinary facility. Systems that would previously fill a pickup truck have been reduced to compact bench-top analyzers. The cost

Dr. Weiser is a shareholder and part-time employee of Heska Corporation. Dr. Vap is a shareholder and intermittent consultant of Abaxis. Dr. Thrall is a part-time employee of Antech Diagnostics.

*Corresponding author. Heska Corporation, 3760 Rocky Mountain Avenue, Loveland, CO 80538. E-mail address: weiserg@heska.com (M.G. Weiser).

0195-5616/07/$ – see front matter
doi:10.1016/j.cvsm.2006.11.005

of acquisition of equivalent capability is approximately 5% or less in inflation-adjusted dollars compared with 20 years ago. The authors predict that this trend to deliver increased diagnostic capability to point of care facilities is going to continue. In future systems, predicted trends in diagnostic instrumentation systems include reduced complexity, increased reliability through self-monitoring, improved information management capability, and improved connectivity with hospital databases within practice management software.

The veterinary and human laboratory diagnostic settings are not equal, however, creating some basic concerns about diagnostic instrumentation making its way to the veterinary market. Currently, it is the responsibility of the veterinary community to manage these concerns in the implementation of laboratory technology for improved veterinary patient care. The concerns may be summarized as follows. Diagnostic instrumentation is offered to the human medical market with a few assumptions that are not true for the veterinary market. The first concern is governmental regulation. Devices must be approved by the US Food and Drug Administration (FDA) for use in the US human health market. In the veterinary market, however, there is no regulatory or registration requirement. This means that the device may be offered with application claims that are not independently tested or evaluated. The individual veterinarian is at a technical disadvantage to perform evaluations and frankly does not have the time. Second, the devices are designed for users with considerable education in laboratory science and medical technology. Operators in the veterinary setting usually do not have this background and experience; this can lead to suboptimal use or misuse of the devices. Users often do not understand the capabilities and, more importantly, the limitations of these systems. Fortunately, there is movement to formulate more continuing education programs in laboratory technology for animal health technicians. The third concern is system monitoring by a program of quality control. Quality control programs are mandated in human health laboratories, regardless of size. In the veterinary market, however, devices are represented with highly variable to nonexistent quality control programs. The fourth concern is daily testing volume. These systems are designed to handle sample throughput that far exceeds the testing volume in the veterinary facility. Some facilities acquire this diagnostic capability and then only use it for one to two patients per day. The authors' view is that the capital investment, internal educational effort, and proper maintenance of expertise for a relatively sophisticated internal laboratory are not warranted for this testing volume. A recommendation is that the threshold of an average of five patients per day should be considered the minimum to make the in-clinic laboratory endeavor logistically and cost-effective. Those facilities that implement wellness and preanesthetic diagnostics should be able to achieve that volume.

With that background, the purposes of this article are as follows:

1. To review the general technologies available today
2. To provide some guidelines for success in implementation of an in-clinic laboratory

3. To provide some criteria for system evaluation and expectations for comparative performance
4. To review preventive measures for some of the common problems and limitations associated with in-clinic laboratory diagnostics

OVERVIEW OF SYSTEMS AVAILABLE FOR IN-CLINIC LABORATORY DIAGNOSTICS

Similar to a surgical instrument, the veterinarian must understand the capabilities and limitations of the diagnostic laboratory instruments in use to make appropriate diagnostic decisions. The term *instrument* is not used loosely. In the clinical laboratory setting, instruments are used to make precise measurements. A "machine," conversely, is used to make something or to move dirt. The following section describes measuring principles used by several types of instrument systems. Understanding these basic concepts of methodology is a crucial step toward maximizing their utility. Examples of currently available systems are mentioned. For available systems and suppliers, please refer to exhibitor lists at local or regional veterinary meetings for more current or changing information. Pricing information is not addressed here because of rapidly changing information and bundle offerings that may confuse pricing information.

Hematology

Centrifugation

A centrifugal hematology analyzer utilizes a method to make quantitative measurements on cell layers below and within the buffy coat. An example of this technology is Becton Dickinson's quantitative buffy coat (QBC) VetAutoread (Idexx Laboratories, Portland, Maine) [1–4]. As the descriptive name implies, it uses a tube similar to an enlarged microhematocrit capillary tube containing a cylindric float to expand the buffy coat layer further. Granulocytes (neutrophils, eosinophils, and basophils), mononuclear cells (lymphocytes and monocytes), erythrocytes, and platelets are separated into layers based on relative density on centrifugation of anticoagulated whole blood. The tube is placed in a reader, and fluorescent staining differentiates the cell layers. The thickness of each layer provides information for estimating various concentrations. The eosinophil concentration can be estimated in canine and bovine samples, and reticulocyte percentages can be determined in canine and feline samples. Fibrinogen concentration can be determined after incubating the processed sample tube in a precipitator and then spinning and reading it again. For erythrocytes, only the hematocrit is measured. From the hematocrit, hemoglobin and mean cell hemoglobin concentration are estimated assuming a constant relation between these values.

Because individual cells are not analyzed, estimated counts must be obtained by assuming an average cell size. Because the erythrocyte count is not determined, mean cell volume (MCV) cannot be calculated. Platelet sizes vary depending on the level of regeneration and may affect the accuracy when low numbers of large platelets are present.

Impedance

Impedance analyzers use the Coulter principle to analyze individual cells. The principle is based on cells being relatively poor electrical conductors in a surrounding conductive electrolyte solution. Electrodes are present on either side of a small aperture through which the cells pass, typically individually. A change in voltage is measured with each passage and provides for a volumetric assessment of each cell. The number of voltage changes indicates cell numbers, and the magnitude of change reflects the cell size (volume). Species-specific electronic thresholds are set to exclude cells and debris falling outside a desired size range. The systems use a precise volume and dilution of sample; thus, concentration can be determined. As a result, impedance methodology can provide relatively reliable and accurate information related to leukocyte, erythrocyte, and platelet concentrations and size distributions. Erythrocyte and platelet indices, including MCV, red cell distribution width (RDW), and mean platelet volume (MPV), can be calculated or derived from the measurements obtained.

Impedance analyzers typically aspirate the sample and then divide and dilute the portions in isotonic fluid. One dilution is exposed to a reagent that lyses erythrocytes to prevent them from interfering with leukocyte determinations and to allow for the hemoglobin concentration measurement by spectrophotometry. A second isotonic dilution retains cellular integrity for erythrocyte and platelet determinations. In this dilution, a threshold excludes leukocytes from other cell populations based on their large size and low relative concentration. Platelets and erythrocytes are separable for clinical interpretation purposes by thresholds.

Three-part differentials are obtained that include granulocytes, lymphocytes, and monocytes. Cells are differentiated by the size of nuclear material and cell remnants after treatment with a reagent that minimizes or removes the cytoplasmic membrane. When viewing the histogram, granulocytes appear as the largest cells, lymphocytes as the smallest, and monocytes fall in between. Nucleated erythrocytes are included with lymphocytes or monocytes depending on their maturity level and size of their nucleus. Examples of analyzers using impedance technology include the HM series (Abaxis, Union City, California), the CBC-Diff system (Heska Corporation, Loveland, Colorado), the AcT analyzer with veterinary software (Beckman Coulter, Fullerton, California), and the HemaVet 950 analyzer (Drew Scientific, Oxford, Connecticut). The HemaVet 950 incorporates "focused flow" and conductivity, along with the impedance measurement; as a result, a five-part differential is claimed. Although the use of impedance technology is long and well investigated in the human literature, recently published comparison data are scarce for impedance-based analyzers using veterinary samples [5,6].

Light scatter

Light scatter involves a sample stream encased in a column of sheath fluid so that cells are passed by the laser light source in single file. Light is deflected off the cells based on size and internal makeup. Forward, right-angle, and side-angle light scatter is measured by photodetectors and is used to distinguish and evaluate the various cell populations. Low-angle scatter is related to cell size. Erythrocytes are lysed to prevent interference with leukocyte evaluations, and hemoglobin is measured by spectrophotometry. Neutrophils and eosinophils produce higher angle light scatter than other leukocytes based on their granularity; thus, a five-part differential is claimed.

Several analyzers use variations of the laser or light scatter method [7–11]. The LaserCyte (Idexx Laboratories) uses light scatter alone. The primary advantage of light scatter systems is additional information to obtain five-part leukocyte differentiation. The consistency of leukocyte differentiation in animals is not ideal, however, resulting in most laboratories continuing to perform microscopy differentials on all samples. The differential from light scatter systems is most applicable to toxicology laboratories that deal with large numbers of normal samples.

The Cell-Dyn 3500 (Abbott Laboratories, Abbott Park, Illinois) and XE-2100 (Sysmex America, Mundelein, Illinois) use varying proprietary approaches to light scatter analysis combined with impedance technology. The Advia 120 (Bayer Diagnostics, Tarrytown, New Jersey) uses light scatter combined with peroxidase cytochemistry. Some systems, such as the Advia 120, also provide some advanced erythrocyte subpopulation indices that are likely to prove useful with additional clinical experience. These systems are inherently more complex and costly and are more appropriate for high-volume clinical laboratories and research support laboratories [12].

Clinical Chemistry
Liquid chemistry systems
Liquid chemistry analyzers are the most traditional chemistry systems and are the type used in most commercial laboratories. After addition of sample to a liquid reagent mixture, a chemical reaction occurs, producing development of a reactant with a specific color in the reaction mixture. Light of a specific wavelength is passed through the mixture. A photodetector measures the development of color change, which is proportional to the concentration of the analyte or enzyme activity. Systems may incorporate blanking methods to minimize interference from hemolysis, lipemia, or icterus; however, the user should be aware of when such interference exists. This may be aided by the reporting of numeric values related to these sample quality issues. These systems tend to have the greatest flexibility in test selection allowing for customized panels. Reagent use management is complex, however. In general, the complexity of these systems and associated reagent management make them unsuitable for the typical in-clinic laboratory.

Dry chemistry systems
Dry reagent systems use reflectance photometry. Reagent test strips are impregnated with chemistry reagents in a dried form. Sample reconstitutes the reagents and triggers development of color reactions in a reaction layer.

Sample is applied with manual or automated pipetting to a reaction pad or multilayered reaction slide, a reaction occurs, and a photometer measures the amount of light reflected from the surface. The test strips can have one to multiple reaction pads, allowing for individualized and defined panel testing. Panel testing is accomplished with dry slide systems by loading desired slides into the testing unit. These typically include the common chemistry analytes but not electrolytes [13]. Advantages include simple reagent use management; flexibility for user-defined test menus; and minimal interference from hemolysis, lipemia, and icterus. Examples of systems using this methodology include the SPOTCHEM (Heska Corporation), VetTest (Idexx Laboratories), and Reflo-Vet Plus (scil Animal Care Company, Grayslake, Illinois) analyzers.

Reconstituted liquid chemistry systems
Analyzers using reconstituted liquid, such as the VetScan (Abaxis) and Hemagen Analyst (Hemagen Diagnostics, Columbia, Maryland), are similar to liquid analyzers except that the reagents are in lyophilized form and are physically separated into individual chambers in a rotor device. The rotor is designed to distribute sample to the reagent chambers, whereby it reconstitutes reagents for measurement reaction. Centrifugal force is used to mix the sample with the reagent(s). The chemical reactions typically occur in individualized reaction chambers placed on a rotor that double as cuvettes. A spectrophotometer is used to measure the reaction similar to that of liquid analyzers. The rotor system allows for the most simple reagent use management, and test menus are fixed by the rotor configuration. The VetScan allows the use of heparinized whole blood.

Electrochemistry
Electrochemistry involves the measurement of electrical potential difference (potentiometry) or generated current (amperometry) in chemical reactions. Common to all types of electrochemistry are the sample, electrodes, a measuring device, membranes, and electrolyte solutions to provide electrical contact between the electrodes. Also known as ion selective electrode technology, electrochemistry is the reference procedure for measurement of ion concentrations. Examples include the common electrolytes, pH, ionized calcium, and blood gas measurements. The principle involves equilibration of ions across a membrane with the exception of the ion being measured. The membrane contains chemistry to exclude equilibration of the ion being measured. This exclusion results in a potential difference across the membrane that is directly related to the concentration of the ion being measured. This potential difference is measured, and the concentration is calculated using the Nernst equation.

Some clinical chemistry measurements may be performed when linked to an enzymatic reaction that generates ions. Hematocrit may also be estimated by resistance to electrical conduction through a whole-blood sample, a principle known as conductometry.

Examples of blood gas and electrolyte analyzers include the IRMA blood analysis system (ITC, Edison, New Jersey), i-STAT system (Heska

Corporation), VetLyte and VetStat analyzers (Idexx Laboratories), and Easy-Lyte Plus (Hemagen Diagnostics). Advantages include the ability to measure analytes not available by other means, and for urgent care testing, whole blood may be used.

GUIDELINES FOR SUCCESS IN IMPLEMENTATION OF AN IN-CLINIC LABORATORY

Selection of Instrumentation and Supplier for In-Clinic Laboratory Support

Instrumentation selection is perceived by most as confusing and by some as risky. A typical checklist of considerations might include the following:

- Ease of use and ease of learning to use the system
- Reputation for reliability and accuracy. Other than anecdotal perceptions from colleagues, this is often difficult information to obtain.
- A corollary to reliability is whether the system comes with a reasonable quality control program that monitors the ability to recover results from some consistent standard.
- Diagnostic menu capability. Does it meet the needs for intended use? Most systems provide menus suitable for wellness and preanesthetic diagnostics as well as a basic screening laboratory database for sick animal patients.
- Patient report style(s) and ease of use for data interpretation and as client communication tools
- Expectations for communication with practice management patient databases
- Performance evaluation data. Ask the supplier for any independent or internal data on reproducibility and comparison with a standard. Unfortunately, these kinds of evaluations are not frequently done.
- Performance evaluation on a trial basis. Veterinarians are inclined to perform their own performance evaluation. This usually boils down to perception rather than an appropriate evaluation based on data. People typically analyze a few samples that are split and sent to a commercial laboratory. They often have unrealistic expectations about comparison of results and do not come to valid conclusions. The simplest way to evaluate a system rapidly is to perform a reproducibility test. This involves a single sample analyzed repetitively 10 to 20 times. The values of interest are then put into a table in which one can inspect the spread of results from minimum to maximum. Does the variation meet your expectations for clinical interpretation purposes? A general guideline is that on an individual system, the reproducibility should be considerably tighter than the assay value limit range for the same measurement in a quality control program sample (see the section on understanding expectations for reproducibility and interlaboratory comparison). If the system cannot achieve satisfactory reproducibility, it inherently cannot achieve accuracy. If good reproducibility can be documented, accuracy may be ensured by recovery of quality control values that are tied to reference procedures. Generally, chemistry systems have satisfactory to excellent performance. For hematology, performance is much more variable as a result of how dilutions are made and processed in fluidic systems.

- Cost-effectiveness of the operation for the predicted testing volume
- Patient sample volume requirements, counter space and consumable storage requirements, and portability for ambulatory applications may be user-specific considerations.
- Communication between the supplier and user. When considering the purchase of diagnostic instrumentation, one is not making an isolated capital equipment purchase. One is entering into an ongoing relationship and depends on introductory training, a consumable supply stream, technical support, and service support. It is also important that the supplier be able to offer or advise on ancillary sample handling and preparation aids.

User Group

In any given busy practice setting, there may be numerous users of the diagnostic instrumentation. Use is typically delegated to the animal health technician staff by the veterinarian(s). Technicians often come in and out of the use picture and may receive variable training specific to the systems being used. The problems associated with this are commonly compounded by the lack of user education and experience in laboratory technology. When there are inaccurate patient results, it is almost always associated with misuse of the technology rather than with failure of the technology. To prevent this kind of user failure and to achieve optimal performance of the laboratory, it is recommended that a single person be designated as the lead technologist for the endeavor. This is often known as "key operator" status in laboratory settings. This person should have a strong interest in laboratory diagnostics and be allocated time to take on this responsibility. A checklist of responsibilities for this role should include the following:

- Thoroughly read and refer to user manuals. Pose questions to supplier technical support whenever there is operational uncertainty.
- Be familiar with sample handling recommendations and procedures provided by the supplier.
- Oversee the quality control program(s) (see the article by Weiser and Thrall found elsewhere in this issue).
- Schedule and monitor performance of recommended periodic maintenance procedures. This should include daily startup and shutdown procedures, associated cleaning, and simple service that may be required as follow-up to troubleshooting.
- Be the primary contact with supplier technical support for troubleshooting.
- Develop a training checklist for education of other users in the facility. This should include sample handling and operation of the system(s).

Attention to Detail

It is critical that everyone in the diagnostic events chain rigorously adhere to principles and supplier recommendations for laboratory testing procedures. This includes animal preparation before sample collection, proper anticoagulant use and sample handling after collection, and sample handling specific to the instrumentation being used. Some principles common to most or all systems are outlined in the next section. This should be supplemented by more specific information from the supplier.

Understanding Expectations for Reproducibility, Interlaboratory Comparison of Results, and Changes in Laboratory Results Over Time

Some users get frustrated when laboratory results are inconsistent with preconceived notions or seem "different" from results obtained from a commercial laboratory. If a single sample is analyzed repeatedly on the same system, there is an expected degree of variation from result to result. That variation inherently increases if multiple analyzers of the same type are used for the measurements. If different methods or systems are used for comparative measurements, the variation increases yet further, sometimes dramatically. Typically, large differences imposed by different methods have different reference ranges. When users do not understand the acceptable magnitude of these differences, they may make false conclusions about a system's accuracy or undertake unnecessary troubleshooting. This is one value of a quality control program—to provide assurance that the system is recovering a standardized value for a known sample measurement (see the article by Weiser and Thrall found elsewhere in this issue).

The following is intended to set expectations for variation that may occur for various chemistry and hematology measurements. The Clinical Laboratory Improvement Amendments (CLIA) established in 1988 are used to regulate human health laboratory testing in the United States. There are CLIA guidelines outlining the proficiency expectation for acceptable variability in laboratory test results [14]. On the basis of these guidelines, some examples of expected variation in results were constructed for hematology (Table 1) and clinical chemistry (Table 2). Results are shown first for a family of the same instrument type. These results may be used as a reproducibility target for an in-house analyzer. Typically, a single in-house instrument is expected to be

Table 1
Expectations for variability in laboratory test results; hematology

Measurement in sample	Hematocrit (%)	Mean cell volume (fL)	Hemoglobin (g/dL)	Platelets ($\times 10^3/\mu L$)	White blood cells ($\times 10^3/\mu L$)
Example mean target value	40	70	15	300	10,000
CLIA proficiency guideline	±6%	±5%	±7%	±25%	±15%
For same instrument type[a]	37.5–42.5	67–73	14.0–16.0	225–375	8500–11,500
Variation across multiple methods[b]	35–45	65–75	13.2–16.8	200–400	7500–12,500

Abbreviation: CLIA, Clinical Laboratory Improvement Amendments.

[a] Indicates the CLIA proficiency guideline for variation within a large number of identical instruments in the field.

[b] Indicates expected variation for multiple instrument types and methods in a large number of laboratories.

Table 2
Expectations for variability in laboratory test results; clinical chemistry

Measurement in sample	BUN	Creatinine	ALT (IU/L)	ALP (IU/L)	Phos	Bilirubin	Calcium	Glucose	Tpro (g/L)	Albumin (g/dl)
Example mean target value	50	6.9	135	326	7.3	7.2	13.0	300	4.6	2.1
CLIA proficiency guideline	±9%	±15%	±20%	±30%	±10%	±20%	±1.0 mg/dL	±10%	±10%	±10%
For same instrument type[a]	45–55	5.9–7.9	110–160	228–423	6.6–8.0	5.8–8.6	12.0–14.0	270–330	4.1–5.1	1.9–2.3
Variation across multiple methods[b]	33–62	4.7–10.0	70–160	185–500	5.8–8.8	4.7–9.1	11.2–15.0	240–389	3.0–5.8	1.3–2.7

Units are mg/dl unless otherwise indicated.
Abbreviations: ALP, alkaline phosphatase; ALT, alanine aminotransferase; BUN, blood urea nitrogen; CLIA, Clinical Laboratory Improvement Amendments; Phos, inorganic phosphorus; Tpro, total protein.
[a]Indicates the CLIA proficiency guideline for variation within a large number of identical instruments in the field.
[b]Indicates expected variation for multiple instrument types and methods in a large number of laboratories.

considerably tighter than a group of identical instruments because of minor variation introduced by multiple systems. At a minimum, however, a single system should not exceed these limits to be considered a system with good performance (see Tables 1 and 2). Cumulative quality control data on in-house analyzers may also provide another measure of reproducibility performance. Variation for instruments and methods of multiple kinds are then shown; these are derived from example quality control data for human laboratories. These results are useful for perspective on how results may differ between an in-house laboratory and a commercial laboratory. The CLIA guidelines typically are expressed as a plus or minus percentage of a mean or true value. Therefore, the magnitude of variation depends on the magnitude of the true value. Most of the examples show variation for abnormal results, which is where a question usually arises. Larger differences are anticipated for measurements like enzyme activities because this kind of measurement is more sensitive to variables than measurement of a concentration (see Table 2).

Instrument manufacturers often provide reproducibility specifications in the form of coefficients of variation (CVs). It is recommended that users not use CV values for reproducibility evaluations. When performing a reproducibility test, it is much more informative to examine the minimum and maximum values. The CV is an industry convention, but it is difficult to interpret the range of variation for clinical interpretation purposes. The unit of the CV is percentage. This does not mean that the results are plus or minus that percentage. Generally, the range of variation for a CV percentage is considerably greater than that percentage.

A corollary to variation in measurements is that users may overinterpret the magnitude of difference in results from two samples taken from the same animal at different points in time. Some are shocked to learn the magnitude of variation that may occur from hour to hour or day to day as a result of biologic response or pathology. It takes a lot of experience to learn which measurements are biologically stable from day to day (an example is erythrocyte MCV) and which may change dramatically (examples include white blood cell [WBC] concentration and many of the chemistry analytes).

A concluding recommendation is to become familiar with reproducibility expectations so that the following may occur:

- Through familiarity with the CLIA guidelines, become more forgiving of differences in measurement results between in-house instrumentation and commercial laboratories by understanding the expected variation that may occur. It may be appropriate to ask about such differences, but avoid the initial conclusion that something is broken.
- When interpreting sequential changes over time, look for changes that exceed expected variation before interpreting them as a biologic response or disease improvement or worsening. In general, it is best to look for large changes before concluding that they represent a meaningful patient response.

SAMPLE HANDLING, PREVENTING COMMON PROBLEMS, AND LIMITATIONS OF DIAGNOSTIC INSTRUMENTATION

Experience indicates that almost all problems with in-house laboratory testing are related to sample handling or procedural misconceptions. It is recommended that the veterinarian, animal health technician, and any other persons involved with in-clinic laboratory testing be familiar with these guidelines in addition to guidelines provided by their supplier.

Hematology

Anticoagulants

Historically, liquid tripotassium (ethylenediaminetetraacetic acid [EDTA]) has been the anticoagulant of choice for hematology system measurements. Reference methods and calibration procedures depended on this EDTA salt to obtain accurate cell volume measurements used to derive the hematocrit. Tubes containing powdered forms of EDTA are discouraged. More recently, dipotassium EDTA spray dried in tubes has been adopted to be more forgiving of user variability in placing the appropriate volume in EDTA tubes. It is predicted that over time, K2 EDTA tubes are likely to replace K3 EDTA for hematologic applications.

It should be noted that lithium heparin samples might give a false high hematocrit by instrument methods and centrifugation, apparently as a result of cell swelling. Hematocrits measured in electrochemical systems by conductometry are reliable with lithium heparin or unanticoagulated whole blood immediately introduced to the analyzer. EDTA or other anticoagulated samples are not appropriate for use in electrochemical devices.

Blood collection and sample handling after collection

When collecting the sample for hematologic analysis, it is important to obtain a clean venipuncture to avoid tissue contamination that can activate platelet aggregation. Platelet clumping in animal blood samples is a common problem. Platelet clumping reduces the measured platelet concentration in hematology analyzers and also traps leukocytes, interfering with that measurement to variable degrees. Worse yet is when platelet clumping is severe enough to cause grossly detectable clots. Aspiration of clots into hematology systems not only gives erroneous results but creates the need for clearance and system cleaning. It may also increase the frequency of maintenance or service procedures. Collection of blood from catheter lines should be avoided because of user errors associated with this procedure. A 20-gauge or larger needle should be used for venipuncture. Extremely small-gauge needles should be avoided because it takes too long to obtain the sample and turbulence increases the chance of hemolysis.

After collection, the blood should be immediately transferred to the EDTA tube. The transfer should be made slowly through the needle or from the syringe with the needle and tube cap removed to avoid hemolysis of the sample. It is then critical to mix the blood tube by gentle inversion several times immediately after filling. The timing and mixing are important to prevent initiation of biochemical clotting reactions.

After collection, the blood should be handled in accordance with the following guidelines:

- Blood should be properly mixed by gentle inversion of the EDTA tube immediately before an aliquot is removed for any procedure. Ideally, this is done with a blood mixing device. The blood may be left on a blood mixing device as soon as it is delivered to the laboratory.
- Analysis on hematology systems should be performed after 10 minutes and before 4 hours after collection. The rationale is that leukocyte differential measurements are most reliable in this interval. Poorly understood equilibration of blood with EDTA may be associated with suboptimal differential performance if blood is analyzed less than 10 minutes after collection.
- The blood tube should be kept at room temperature within the previously mentioned analysis time. If the blood needs to be stored longer than this, it should be stored in the refrigerator. Never allow the blood tube to freeze.
- Air-dried blood films should be prepared at the time of blood collection or within 15 minutes. Blood films should be stored at room temperature.

Understanding limitations of automated differentials and use of blood films
The automated differential is the most important limitation of in-house hematology systems. A common misconception is that cell counters with differential capability were invented to replace examination of blood films and differentials by microscopy. For human and animal hematology, the technology is not capable of reliably performing clinically diagnostic differentials when pathologic findings are present. At best, the technology was invented to reduce the number of microscopy differentials by identifying normal leukocyte distributions not requiring additional follow-up. This is done using criteria established in each laboratory. Most veterinary teaching hospital laboratories routinely perform microscopy differentials on all samples.

It is recommended that a blood film be made, stained, and retained on all patients requiring a complete blood cell count (CBC), regardless of the analytic method used. The blood film may be reviewed as a quality control check of leukocyte and platelet measurement obtained from the analyzer. Furthermore, neutrophilic left shifts, nucleated erythrocytes, large granular lymphocytes, mast cells, and immature cells associated with hematopoietic neoplasia are some leukocyte findings identifiable only by examination of a blood film. In addition, identification of hemoparasites, bacteria, inclusions, erythrocyte morphology, and platelet clumps or giant platelets requires blood film review (see the article by Weiser and Thrall found elsewhere in this issue).

Other sample pathology factors related to hematologic analysis
There are instances in which hemopathology may result in analytic errors that are detected by examination of the blood tube or blood film. These include the following:

- Preanalytic issues, such as insufficient anticoagulant tube filling, hemolysis, insufficient sample mixing, and quality of the blood film, can significantly alter results.

- Extremely large platelets may be misclassified as erythrocytes.
- Platelet clumps are excluded from measurement and may be counted as leukocytes, falsely decreasing the platelet concentration and falsely increasing the WBC concentration. This is a common problem in samples collected from cats, and it may occasionally occur in other species as well.
- Rarely, erythrocytes of select animals or species may be resistant to the lyse reagent and falsely increase the leukocyte count.
- Autoagglutination of erythrocytes, seen frequently in immune-mediated hemolytic anemia, may result in red blood cells (RBCs) being excluded from analysis because of the large size of aggregates. Falsely low RBC and hematocrit values and falsely high mean cell hemoglobin concentration (MCHC) and MCV values can occur.

Clinical Chemistry
Anticoagulants
The classic sample type for clinical chemistry is serum. Serum preparation requires no anticoagulant. The sample tube without anticoagulant is commonly referred to as the "red-top" tube. Blood is allowed to clot to completion. This typically takes approximately 15 minutes. The tube is then centrifuged to pack all cellular elements and clot, leaving a supernatant of serum.

More recently, lithium heparin has been adopted for routine clinical chemistry and is available in various convenient and commercially available collection devices. One common device is the lithium heparin vacuum tube. The advantage of lithium heparin is that the sample may be separated by centrifugation without waiting for clot formation to occur to completion. This allows for faster sample processing in the small laboratory. The resulting supernatant, plasma, is suitable for routine clinical chemistry and electrochemical measurements. There are also specialized syringes that contain "balanced" lithium heparin. This means that the heparin has calcium saturation of weak calcium-binding sites on the heparin molecule, making it ideal for measurement of ionized calcium. These devices are ideal for sample collection for use in urgent care electrochemical analyzers, and the sample may also be used for routine chemistry measurements.

In general, other heparin salts and all other anticoagulants should be avoided for clinical chemistry and electrochemistry in the in-clinic laboratory setting. In particular, manual heparinization of syringes should be avoided for use in electrochemical measurements. This typically results in gross overheparinization, which may cause erroneous measurements in modern microfabricated cartridge electrochemical devices.

Sample factors related to chemical analysis
Interfering substances. There are several factors that may interfere with spectrophotometric measurements of clinical chemistry reactions. The interferences vary from system to system. The user should refer to application sheets or technical support to become familiar with the features and magnitudes of interference specific to the system(s) in use. Common factors are lipemia, hemolysis,

and hyperbilirubinemia or icterus. Lipemia occurs most commonly as a result of not fasting the animal before blood collection. It may also occur pathologically in a variety of metabolic disorders. Hemolysis is almost always attributable to improper sample transfer to blood tubes or to use of a small-gauge needle; it is the most preventable factor. Icterus is the least common factor and is not preventable because it is an inherent pathologic finding in the sample.

Fibrination. When blood is collected in a red-top tube, contact with glass initiates the biochemical clotting cascade reaction, with the end point of converting all sample fibrinogen to fibrin. When the sample is centrifuged, fibrin is separated with cells, leaving harvestable serum as a supernatant. Occasionally, samples do not form fibrin to completion in the 15 minutes before centrifugation. This occurs most frequently in tubes that are cooled soon after collection or are in a relatively cool room-temperature environment. Fibrin that forms after separation of the serum is a viscous material that may occlude pipette tips or otherwise displace fluid volume. This can result in dilution or sample volume errors, leading to erroneous laboratory results. Because fibrin may also occlude tubing in the instrument's sample path, this results in the need for system cleaning or other prescribed maintenance. If fibrination is detected as a recurring problem in the clinical laboratory, it is recommended that samples be incubated in a water bath or incubator block at or near body temperature. This drives fibrination to completion in less than 15 minutes and prevents the problem. An alternative solution to this problem is to adopt a lithium heparin collection device and use plasma instead of serum.

SUMMARY
The typical technologies used in veterinary hematology and biochemical analyzers have been reviewed, along with associated advantages and disadvantages. Guidelines for implementing a successful in-clinic laboratory have been provided, including criteria for system evaluation and expectations for comparative performance evaluations. The more common problems and limitations associated with in-clinic laboratory diagnostics and how best to prevent them have also been discussed. Many of these steps may be compared with the links of a chain; the final result is only as reliable as the weakest link. Sample collection and handling as well as data interpretation are only a part of that chain. If the analyzer link is maintained and utilized properly, it should function as an instrument and is most likely to provide consistently reliable results. If not, however, it may become a machine that may as well be used to move dirt.

References
  [1] Levine RA, Hart AH, Wardlaw SC. Quantitative buffy coat analysis of blood collected from dogs, cats, and horses. J Am Vet Med Assoc 1986;189(6):670–3.
  [2] Papasouliotis K, Cue S, Graham M, et al. Analysis of feline, canine and equine hemograms using the QBC VetAutoread. Vet Clin Pathol 1999;28(3):109–15.

[3] Tasker S, Cripps PJ, Mackin AJ. Evaluation of methods of platelet counting in the cat. J Small Anim Pract 2001;42(7):326–32.

[4] Wegmann D, Hofmann-Lehmann R, Lutz H. Short evaluation of the QBC-Vet Autoread System. Tierarztl Prax 1997;25(2):185–91 [in German].

[5] Dewhurst EC, Crawford E, Cue S, et al. Analysis of canine and feline haemograms using the VetScan HMT analyser. J Small Anim Pract 2003;44(10):443–8.

[6] Schwendenwein I, Jolly M. Automated differentials by an impedance on-site hematology analyzer [abstract]. Vet Clin Pathol 2001;30(3):158.

[7] Dawson H, Hoff B, Grift E, et al. Validation of the Coulter AcT Diff hematology analyzer for analysis of blood of common domestic animals. Vet Clin Pathol 2000;29(4):132–6.

[8] Tvedten HW, Korcal D. Automated differential leukocyte count in horses, cattle, and cats using the Technicon H-1E hematology system. Vet Clin Pathol 1996;25(1):14–22.

[9] Tvedten HW, Wilkins RJ. Automated blood cell counting systems: a comparison of the Coulter S-Plus IV, Ortho ELT-8/DS, Ortho ELT-8/WS, Technicon H-1, and Sysmex E-5,000. Vet Clin Pathol 1988;17(2):47–54.

[10] Malin MJ, Sclafani LD, Wyatt JL. Evaluation of 24-second cyanide-containing and cyanide-free methods for whole blood hemoglobin on the Technicon H*1TM analyzer with normal and abnormal blood samples. Am J Clin Pathol 1989;92(3):286–94.

[11] Fernandes PJ, Modiano JF, Wojcieszyn J, et al. Use of the Cell-Dyn 3500 to predict leukemic cell lineage in peripheral blood of dogs and cats. Vet Clin Pathol 2002;31(4):167–82.

[12] Gaunt SD, Prescott-Mathews JS, King WW, et al. Clinical hematology practices at veterinary teaching hospitals and private diagnostic laboratories. Vet Clin Pathol 1995;24(2):64–7.

[13] Lanevschi A, Kramer JW. Comparison of two dry chemistry analyzers and a wet chemistry analyzer using canine serum. Vet Clin Pathol 1996;25(1):10–3.

[14] Clinical Laboratory Improvement Amendments. CLIA proficiency testing criteria. Fed Regist 1992;57(40):7002–186. Available at: http://www.westgard.com/clia.htm. Accessed December 26, 2006.

Vet Clin Small Anim 37 (2007) 237–244

VETERINARY CLINICS
SMALL ANIMAL PRACTICE

Quality Control Recommendations and Procedures for In-Clinic Laboratories

M. Glade Weiser, DVM[a,b,*], Mary Anna Thrall, DVM, MS[a,c]

[a]Department of Microbiology, Immunology, and Pathology, College of Veterinary Medicine and Biomedical Sciences, Colorado State University, Fort Collins, CO 80523, USA
[b]Heska Corporation, 3760 Rocky Mountain Avenue, Loveland, CO 80538, USA
[c]Department of Pathobiology, Ross University School of Veterinary Medicine, Basseterre, St. Kitts, West Indies

Q uality control monitoring of hematology and clinical chemistry instrumentation diagnostics has been established in clinical and commercial laboratories from their inception. Everyone acknowledges in principle that quality control monitoring also applies to in-clinic laboratory instrumentation. This acknowledgment has been poorly reduced to practice in the veterinary facility, however. The universally recognized necessity for in-clinic quality control in laboratory diagnostics was re-emphasized to the veterinary profession several years ago [1]. The cited publication suggested that quality control procedures used in professional laboratories might be too extensive for the small veterinary facility, but an alternative solution was not provided.

More recently, the Committee for Quality Assurance and Standards of the American Society for Veterinary Clinical Pathology (ASVCP) formulated a comprehensive document for quality control standards applicable to all veterinary laboratories. These are published on the organization's web site [2]. The society is commended for taking a leadership position for formulating these standards in the absence of regulatory oversight of veterinary laboratory testing. In-clinic laboratory endeavors are veterinary laboratories and, as such, should move toward implementation of quality control monitoring.

Lack of regulation in veterinary testing is one factor in quality control monitoring not being well reduced to practice in veterinary hospital facilities. As a result, most users are left to follow recommendations of suppliers of diagnostic instrumentation. Some suppliers state or imply that their respective systems do not require quality control monitoring. Although this may seem expedient and appealing to the user, it is misleading and contrary to ASVCP guidelines.

Dr. Weiser is a shareholder and part-time employee of Heska Corporation. Dr. Thrall is a part-time employee of Antech Diagnostics.

*Corresponding author. Heska Corporation, 3760 Rocky Mountain Avenue, Loveland, CO 80538. E-mail address: weiserg@heska.com (M.G. Weiser).

0195-5616/07/$ – see front matter
doi:10.1016/j.cvsm.2006.11.006

Because of the proliferation of in-clinic laboratory endeavors, it is recommended that the profession, users, and suppliers catch up on implementation of doable quality control monitoring in veterinary facilities. The overall goal here is to demystify implementation of quality control monitoring and encourage increased adoption for laboratory testing in the veterinary hospital.

With that background, the purposes of this article are as follows:

1. To describe the design and use of quality control monitoring material
2. To review the rationale and advantages for quality control monitoring of in-clinic instrumentation
3. To propose a simplified program of quality control monitoring for adoption by the small veterinary laboratory and front-line veterinary medicine
4. To describe hematologic procedures using patient samples that are an adjunct to the quality control program
5. To mention the role of interlaboratory proficiency testing programs
6. To provide an example of an exception

QUALITY CONTROL MONITORING MATERIAL DESIGN AND USE

Control samples are designed to be similar to and analyzed like patient samples. They must also have a reasonable shelf life and open vial stability. To achieve that combination of features, the materials may be treated in ways that are part of the art of creating these products. For clinical chemistry, the material starts with pooled serum in which analytes may be spiked to achieve desired concentrations. For hematology, the erythrocytes are from pooled whole blood. The platelets and leukocytes are not stable and are not present in the material. Other particles are added to mimic leukocytes and platelets in hematology controls.

Once these materials are prepared to create a "lot," they are assayed by reference procedures to establish known concentrations or measurements that are indexed to standards. The materials are then assayed on carefully maintained instruments of the type supported in the field. These data are used to define lot-specific target assay ranges for the instrument type being supported. The limits of assay value ranges are defined by statistical treatment of data from a relatively large number of repetitive analyses on the instrument system. These limits are designed to accommodate the variation that is expected to exist in a family of the same instrument type. These limits should be similar to the Clinical Laboratory Improvement Amendments (CLIA) guidelines for acceptable variability presented in the article by Weiser and colleagues found elsewhere in this issue. The user's individual analyzer range performance from day to day is likely tighter than the assay ranges.

For the user, it is critical that control materials have assay values specific for the analyzer type and method being used. For example, one cannot use a material having assay values for analyzer type X and use it for analyzer type Y. It is possible for a laboratory to obtain a control material and develop its own assay values, but these procedures are not recommended for the typical in-clinic laboratory. As a result, the best source of control material and program is from the supplier supporting the user's instrument.

The logistics of the in-house control program in the facility are as follows. Analysis of control material is performed on a regular basis once per day at the startup of daily patient sample testing. Each day, the results of analysis are checked by inspection against the target assay value ranges. The goal is documentation that the system is recovering the values within the assay value range. Because the assay value ranges can usually be entered into the system software, the user interface may be used to simplify this inspection with a system of results flagging. The system or attached computer system should also accumulate the daily quality control data so that the data are available for trend inspection or submission to technical support if needed. Finally, the control material may be spot-analyzed at any time that the system is questioned or if patient results are questioned.

The user may encounter quality control values that fall outside the assay limits. Following are some action guidelines for this occurrence, but, ultimately, action should be directed by the specific user manual and supplier technical support.

- It is anticipated that an occasional measurement may fall barely outside the assay limits. For most programs, there is approximately a 1% probability of this occurring. This does not require action if it is an isolated incident and the value returns to the assay limit range on the next control sample analysis. Some laboratories immediately repeat a control sample when a value is barely out of range.
- If a measurement or set of measurements is clearly falling outside the assay limits by an appreciable magnitude, action should be taken to determine the cause. Action should be based on specific instructions for a system as defined in its user manual and additional information provided by the supplier.
- It may be noticed that a certain measurement or set of measurements consistently runs near the lower or upper assay limit. This is an indication that the system may be in need of calibration to move the measurements toward the control program mean value. Any action should be based on specific instructions for a system as defined in its user manual and additional information provided by the supplier.

RATIONALE AND ADVANTAGES OF QUALITY CONTROL MONITORING IN HEMATOLOGY AND CLINICAL CHEMISTRY

Technical Perspective

From the technical perspective, laboratory instrumentation performs a complex series of activities, such as automated pipetting, dilutions, mixing, measurements involving current or light, and data reduction. Components like tubing, valves, printed circuit boards, and moving parts are subject to deterioration and eventual failure. Any developing defect or failure in such a complex electromechanical system has an impact on the integrity of final laboratory test results that the system generates. Quality control monitoring was invented to detect this impact on laboratory test results before putting the data into use by the clinician. This has been the objective of daily quality control monitoring programs being implemented as standard operating procedure in clinical laboratories. Daily quality control monitoring programs should be implemented as standard operating procedure in clinical laboratories, regardless of size. Regular use of a control sample ensures that the system is performing to specification in its ability to recover values of the sample with known values anchored to reference procedures.

Clinician's Perspective

From the clinical perspective, a quality control program enables the clinician to interpret laboratory data with greater confidence. Clinicians are frequently presented with laboratory test results that are surprising or not in keeping with preconceived expectations for a given case. This inherently raises questions about the accuracy of those results. A daily quality control monitoring program provides a day-to-day confidence level that patient results have a high probability of being reliable. In addition, the daily quality control program provides the following benefits:

- The daily program is pre-emptive of inefficient and frustrating after-the-fact system troubleshooting with controls only after patient results are questioned. This is particularly difficult if there are no control materials on hand.
- Examination of historical quality control data, generally the last 20 to 30 days, along with a current control sample is an essential first step in instrument troubleshooting when a problem does occur. This is highly valuable for interacting with the supplier's technical support.
- The cumulative quality control data are a source of information for evaluating the system's reproducibility performance over time.
- Most think that the value of quality control is to detect the occasional occurrence of a system problem. It is proposed that the peace of mind associated with documenting the absence of a problem on a daily basis is of greater value.

PROPOSED APPROACH TO SMALL LABORATORY QUALITY CONTROL MONITORING

To date, there has not been uniform treatment of the question of what constitutes a reasonable quality control program for the in-clinic veterinary laboratory. Models of quality control programs exist in human medical laboratories. These are a result of regulation. Most large veterinary laboratories have adopted these guidelines without rethinking them. Standard laboratory guidelines call for analysis of control materials each laboratory shift. Control programs also typically consist of three levels for hematology, known as low, normal, and high, and two levels for clinical chemistry, known as normal and abnormal. Laboratories may insert additional control samples throughout the day when running large numbers of samples. This may result in 5 to 10 or considerably more quality control analyses for hematology and clinical chemistry per day. These guidelines are daunting for the in-clinic veterinary laboratory. This not only consumes considerable time and consumables, but the evaluation of that much data is disproportionately difficult for the objective being considered.

The following is the rationale for a recommended streamlined approach to make quality control monitoring more efficient and palatable for the in-clinic laboratory endeavor. The genesis of multiple levels of control was related to an era when method and instrument linearity was variable and less than ideal. Over the years, there has been marked improvement in measurement dynamic range and linearity. As a result, it is proposed that a multiple-level control program is an obsolete concept for small clinical laboratories. It is also a vestige of large laboratory programs as a result of regulation that is slow to reinvent historical procedures.

It is therefore recommended that single-level controls are adequate for in-house veterinary laboratories. For hematology, this should be the normal level or midrange control. For clinical chemistry, this should be the high or abnormal level control because some analytes, such as bilirubin, are near zero in the normal-level material. The frequency of quality control analysis is recommended to be once each working day for reasons discussed previously. This is also adequate for the in-house veterinary laboratory.

In summary, a program of one control sample per working day for each hematology and chemistry analyzer is efficient, economic, and quite doable for the in-clinic laboratory. It is recommended that the profession and suppliers work together to achieve this kind of program tailored to the needs of in-clinic veterinary laboratories.

HEMATOLOGIC PROCEDURES THAT ARE A SUPPLEMENT TO THE QUALITY CONTROL PROGRAM

There are a couple of tools that may be applied to patient samples to verify analyzer performance on individual samples. One tool is the blood film, as described in the article by Weiser and colleagues found elsewhere in this issue. The other important and underutilized tool is the mean cell hemoglobin concentration (MCHC) value.

Blood Film Review

As mentioned in the article by Weiser and colleagues found elsewhere in this issue, the blood film is an essential quality adjunct to verification of selected platelet and leukocyte measurements. This requires use of a good-quality microscope and well-prepared blood films. Detailed descriptions of blood film examination are delegated to textbooks of veterinary clinical pathology. Some examples of verifications include the following:

- If the analyzer produces an extremely low or extremely high cell concentration, it is easy to verify that result by scanning the blood film with low magnification. For an extremely low cell concentration, leukocytes are rare to absent on the blood film. Conversely, for an extremely high concentration, the leukocyte density is increased compared with normal.

- For patients with abnormal leukocyte concentrations or distributions within the differential, it is important to verify these by a microscopy differential. In these situations, analytic systems may misclassify cells. Also, analytic systems do not identify or classify bands, toxic change, mast cells, or abnormal cells in leukemic states. As a result, many veterinary laboratories routinely perform microscopy differentials and do not report instrument differentials.
- When platelet concentration is decreased on an analyzer measurement, it is important to verify this by scanning the blood film for platelet microclots that may result in a false low measurement.

Mean Cell Hemoglobin Concentration Value

The MCHC value has minimal clinical usefulness but is a highly useful system quality control tool in real-time analysis of patient samples. The rationale is as follows. The MCHC is calculated from the hematocrit (HCT) and hemoglobin concentration values. Within common domestic animal species, the MCHC value is a physiologic constant (typically ranging from 32–38 g/dL) that may be used to monitor the relation between the hemoglobin concentration and HCT. The HCT and hemoglobin concentration are measured in completely separate blood dilutions and analytic subsystems. If there is a system malfunction in either of the dilutions or subsystem measurements, it may be reflected in the MCHC value. Because these are independent measurements, the hemoglobin value corroborates the HCT value, and vice versa, for each sample. There are also a few pathologic sample conditions that result in MCHC abnormalities. On instrument systems that measure HCT and hemoglobin concentration directly, MCHC abnormalities may be considered in the following way.

Low mean cell hemoglobin concentration

There is no pathologic condition that results in a severe decrease in the MCHC. Extreme erythrocyte regeneration (eg, >25% reticulocytes) may be associated with MCHC values in the range from 29 g/dL to normal. Historically, a decreased MCHC has been associated with iron deficiency anemia. With modern analytic instruments, however, erythrocyte sizing measurements and blood film morphology are much more sensitive for detecting erythrocyte changes associated with iron deficiency. An MCHC between 29 and 32 g/dL should not be interpreted as indicative of iron deficiency without corroborating changes in erythrocyte volume abnormalities, blood film changes, and serum iron biochemistry. MCHC values less than 28 g/dL suggest the high probability of a system problem that should be evaluated with blood controls and supplier-recommended troubleshooting. The same is true for MCHC values in the range of 28 to 32 g/dL if this is reasonably consistent across multiple patient samples.

High mean cell hemoglobin concentration

An MCHC value that exceeds 38 g/dL should prompt review of a checklist of pathologic conditions that may cause this. This list includes the following:

- Increased turbidity in the hemoglobin measurement by spectrophotometry. Known causes are lipemia (most common), a high concentration of large

Heinz bodies in cats, and extreme leukocytosis (typically >150,000 per microliter).
- Marked sample hemolysis such that preanalytic lysis of erythrocyte results in a false low HCT.
- Erythrocyte agglutination that does not disperse in the dilution in which the HCT is measured. The HCT is falsely decreased because agglutinated erythrocytes are not included in the measurement. The hemoglobin measurement is accurate. This occurs frequently in immune-mediated hemolytic anemia.

Once the causes on this checklist are ruled out and there is an unexplainable high MCHC, attention should turn to evaluation of the instrument system with controls. In particular, if high MCHCs are occurring across multiple samples, the instrument system should be evaluated for proper function. MCHC values that bounce around sporadically for no apparent reason are an indication of poor system reproducibility. This is also important because leukocytes are measured in the same dilution as hemoglobin.

COMMENTS ON INTERLABORATORY QUALITY CONTROL PROGRAMS

Relatively early in the evolution of professional human and veterinary clinical laboratories, interlaboratory control programs were established to assess how individual laboratories compared with a large number of other laboratories in analysis of an aliquot of the same sample. One historical advantage of this program is that it provided considerable perspective on how much variation could be expected between laboratories for common laboratory tests. Diagnostics companies and laboratory organizations administered these programs.

Laboratories participate in the program three to four times per year, usually quarterly. The administering entity distributes aliquots of a single sample to each subscribing laboratory. Laboratories then analyze the sample and return results for analysis. The laboratory subsequently receives a statistical report indicating how its result compares with a mean value and dispersion based on results from all laboratories.

Some years ago, the Veterinary Laboratory Association (VLA) initiated such a program for veterinary laboratories. Most commercial laboratories, veterinary teaching hospitals, and some research laboratories participate in this program.

Few veterinary hospitals participate in an interlaboratory quality control program. At this point in time, this is not likely to change. This is attributable mostly to the lack of education and awareness about in-clinic quality control programs in general. In addition, it is not recommended without widespread adoption for the following reasons. First, it would take most or a large critical mass of veterinary hospital facilities to subscribe simultaneously to achieve interpretable comparison. This is because in-clinic laboratories are using different instrumentation and methods compared with large laboratories enrolled in the program. Second, an interlaboratory program is not a substitute for an internal program of regular quality control monitoring. Once per quarter is too low a frequency for there to be value in determining if a system problem exists. Therefore, interlaboratory programs are only a supplement to a daily internal quality control program. This may change in the future if a supplier offers its user group a similar program in which the users may compare their results with other users in the same instrument family. As implied in this section, the profession is encouraged to attain a simple interlaboratory comparison program that is tailored to its needs.

AN EXCEPTION

There is at least one blood testing system that is a unique exception to these principles and recommendations (i-STAT analyzer; Heska Corporation, Loveland, Colorado). The design of the system is such that it is not compatible with the use of conventional quality control monitoring programs because the system is, in effect, a new instrument each time a sample is analyzed. The instrument does not pipette sample, makes no dilutions, and has no tubing to age. It uses disposable cartridges that contain microfabricated housing of reference solution, sample chambers, ion selective membranes, and electrodes for electrochemical measurements. The instrument reads electrical signals from the cartridge. For each cycle, it performs a series of electronic checks on cartridge performance, electrical contact, and sample loading. Any defect in cartridge or electronic performance is detected and messaged along with blockage of results reporting. One can run a control sample on a cartridge, but when the next sample is analyzed, it is on a new instrument because all the conventional sample analysis components are housed in the next cartridge. Cartridge performance is quality controlled at the point of manufacturing. The user may run controls to facilitate learning how to use the system and verify recovery of expected results, but this does not control user ability to handle whole-blood samples from patients properly. A batch or lot of cartridges may also be evaluated with controls if shipping or storage conditions have been violated or are otherwise in question. There are likely to be other diagnostic devices in the future with a design that is not amenable to conventional quality control monitoring.

SUMMARY

The design and use of quality control materials and rationale for implementation of a quality monitoring program have been discussed. A simplified approach to a quality monitoring program suitable for in-clinic laboratories has been presented. Use of blood films and the MCHC value as adjuncts to quality monitoring in hematology has been described. Over time, it is hoped that the profession more widely embraces, if not demands, implementation of quality monitoring for in-clinic laboratory diagnostics.

References

[1] Freeman KP, Evans EW, Lester S. Quality control for in-hospital veterinary laboratory testing. J Am Vet Med Assoc 1999;215:928-9.
[2] American Society for Veterinary Clinical Pathology. Quality assurance guidelines. Available at: www.asvcp.org/publications/qas-guidelinemenu.html. Accessed December 26, 2006.

Vet Clin Small Anim 37 (2007) 245–266

VETERINARY CLINICS
SMALL ANIMAL PRACTICE

Hematology Without the Numbers: In-Clinic Blood Film Evaluation

Robin W. Allison, DVM, PhD*,
James H. Meinkoth, DVM, PhD

Department of Veterinary Pathobiology, Center for Veterinary Health Sciences,
Oklahoma State University, 250 McElroy Hall, Stillwater, OK 74078, USA

The complete blood cell count is an integral part of the minimum database. Historically, blood samples were either sent out for analysis to reference laboratories with large, expensive hematology instruments, or were analyzed in-clinic using fairly simple manual methods: a microhematocrit centrifuge and refractometer to determine packed-cell volume and total protein, a hemocytometer to determine the nucleated cell count, and a blood film for the differential leukocyte count. Technical advances and the availability of moderately priced automated hematology instruments are providing more opportunities for private practices to perform rapid in-clinic blood analyses. Although most automated analyzers perform reasonably well with blood samples from normal animals, their performance may be less than optimal with abnormal blood samples from sick animals. One important quality control measure easily accomplished in a short period of time is evaluation of the blood film. Systematic blood film review is essential to confirm the numbers being reported by the hematology instrument, to assess the morphology of erythrocytes and leukocytes, and to look for cell inclusions, hemoparasites, or other microorganisms. The purpose of this article is to outline a simple method of blood film evaluation, highlight the most common clinically important abnormalities that may be seen, and reinforce the importance of blood film evaluation as a quality control measure.

THE PERFECT BLOOD FILM

The quality of the blood film will affect your ability to perform an adequate evaluation. The goal is to produce a blood film with evenly distributed leukocytes in the "counting area" of the film, where the cells are in a monolayer. The basic procedure is known as the *wedge* or *push technique* (see Movie 1 online [within this article at www.vetsmall.theclinics.com, March 2007 issue]).

References to the multimedia components within this article can be found at http://www.theclinics.com, March 2007.

*Corresponding author. E-mail address: robin.allison@okstate.edu (R.W. Allison).

0195-5616/07/$ – see front matter
doi:10.1016/j.cvsm.2006.10.002

A drop of blood is placed near the end of one clean microscope slide. The second slide (pusher slide) is placed in front of the drop of blood at an angle of about 30 to 45 degrees to form a wedge. The pusher slide is backed into the drop of blood; the drop will begin to spread across the bottom edge of the pusher slide. As the drop spreads to almost reach the edges, the pusher slide is rapidly advanced to the end of the first slide. No downward pressure should be used (very important to avoid streaks), and the pusher slide should not be lifted until it is pushed completely off the bottom slide. If downward pressure is difficult to avoid, an alternate method may be useful; the bottom slide can be held flat on the fingers of one hand instead of placed on a tabletop, while the pusher slide is held horizontally by two fingers (see Movie 2 online [within this article at www.vetsmall.theclinics.com, March 2007 issue]). Ideally, the blood film should cover one half to two thirds of the slide, and will be thickest where the drop was placed and get progressively thinner toward the "feathered edge" at the end of the film (Fig. 1). No streaks or gaps should be present because these will affect cell distribution. Preparation of a quality blood film takes some practice, but is an important skill. Varying the speed and angle of the pusher slide will affect the thickness and length of the blood film (higher angle gives a shorter film; slower speed gives a thinner film). Note that samples from very anemic or polycythemic animals may be difficult to work with.

The blood film should be thoroughly dry before staining to prevent water artifact that can distort erythrocytes. This requires letting the blood films sit for at least 5 to 10 minutes, or using a handheld blow dryer in humid environments. For convenience, quick-stain products that mimic the traditional Wright's stain can be used to stain the blood film once it is completely dry. Note that these stains lose strength over time, and need to be changed as necessary for adequate stain quality. They should be completely changed when low, instead of "topping-up" with fresh stain. Stains may also harbor bacteria if not maintained properly, which can create problems when evaluating the blood films.

Blood anticoagulated with ethylenediaminetetraacetic acid (EDTA) is preferred for routine small animal hematology because it does not interfere with cell morphology or staining characteristics. It is important that blood films be made immediately from fresh blood samples to avoid cell-aging changes, which

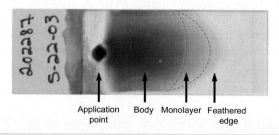

Application   Body   Monolayer   Feathered
point   edge

Fig. 1. A well-made blood film stained with Wright's-Giemsa. The film is thickest at the application point, and becomes progressively thinner toward the feathered edge.

could confuse interpretation; neutrophils develop vacuoles that mimic toxic change, and leukocytes will eventually lyse altogether (Fig. 2). EDTA tubes should be filled to their correct capacity, and blood must be mixed well by gently inverting the tube 10 to 15 times before film preparation to ensure representative cell distribution. Once made, blood films can wait hours or several days to be stained. It is a good idea to make several blood films from each sample; keep the extra slides at room temperature protected from scratches or chemical fumes such as formalin (exposure to formalin fumes prevents adequate cellular staining). If significant or confusing abnormalities are detected, the extra slides can be sent to a reference laboratory or a clinical pathologist for further evaluation.

THE HEMATOLOGY MICROSCOPE

A high-quality microscope is necessary for blood film evaluation; remember that important erythrocyte parasites may be as small as 0.5 μm. Microscopes with high-quality optics are available from a number of different manufacturers for a reasonable price (under $2000). Most of these microscopes come equipped with a set of four objectives: typically 4×, 10×, 40×, and 100× oil immersion. However, a 20× objective can be purchased for a reasonable cost and is recommended for routine hematology because the 40× objective requires a coverslipped slide for sharp focus. A 50× oil immersion objective is also available; it is expensive, but highly utilized by clinical pathologists and other professional microscopists. The light source should have a rheostat to control light intensity. The substage condenser should be raised and the iris diaphragm opened when viewing hematology slides.

APPROACH TO BLOOD FILM EVALUATION

It is important to develop a systematic approach that allows thorough but efficient evaluation of all three cellular components: platelets, erythrocytes, and leukocytes. With practice, most blood films can be thoroughly reviewed in only a few minutes. One suggested approach is shown in Box 1.

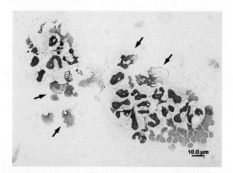

Fig. 2. Marked aging changes in neutrophils. Neutrophils have swollen, pale nuclei and vacuolated basophilic cytoplasm. Arrows indicate cells that have lysed.

Box 1: Approach to blood film evaluation

10× objective

Briefly scan the entire slide, noting the following:

1. Are cells distributed into three recognizable zones (feathered edge, counting area or monolayer, and body of the film or thick area)? The monolayer is identified as the area where erythrocytes are close together but not overlapping. In canine blood, erythrocyte central pallor should be visible in this area. As cells approach the feathered edge they become distorted and flattened, losing their central pallor, and are distributed in an uneven manner.

2. Note the overall thickness of the blood film. Animals that have significant anemia will have thin films, with a very wide and thin counting area. Dehydrated or polycythemic animals will have thick films.

3. Are the leukocytes distributed evenly in the monolayer, or are many cells pulled out to the feathered edge? If cells are not well-distributed, differential counts and estimated cell counts will be inaccurate; a new blood film should be prepared.

4. Look for agglutination of erythrocytes in the body of the film and notice how much rouleaux is present in the monolayer.

5. Check the entire feathered edge of the film for platelet clumps, large abnormal cells, and heartworm microfilaria.

20× objective

1. Estimate the nucleated cell count in the monolayer area of the blood film. A rough estimate can be made by counting the number of nucleated cells per average 20× objective field and multiplying by 500. For example, if there is an average of 20 nucleated cells per 20× objective field in the monolayer, the estimated total nucleated cell count is 10,000/μL. The estimate should roughly approximate the nucleated cell count generated by manual or automated methods. With practice one can quickly assign the cell count to one of three categories: decreased, close to normal, or increased; this is often all that is required for clinical interpretation or quality control.

2. Predict the differential count. Scan the leukocytes to see what cell type appears to predominate, if there are any immature neutrophils present, and if there are large or atypical cells present. Notice if nucleated red blood cells (nRBCs) are present in significant numbers.

3. Note any platelet clumps that you didn't see with the 10× objective.

100× oil immersion objective

Systematically evaluate all three major cell lines in the blood film monolayer: platelets, erythrocytes, and leukocytes.

1. Estimate platelet numbers by counting the number of platelets in several random high power fields. A minimum of 8 to 10 platelets per high power fields should be seen to interpret the numbers as adequate. One platelet per high power fields corresponds roughly to 15,000 to 20,000 platelets per μL. Note enlarged or giant platelets if present (larger than a red cell). Note that the estimated platelet count will be falsely decreased if platelet clumps are present.

2. Note any important erythrocyte shape or color changes, or presence of red cell inclusions or parasites.

3. Perform the differential cell count. For samples with near normal leukocyte numbers, count 100 cells. If leukocytosis is present, count at least 200 cells. Presence of nRBCs can be handled in one of two ways: either included in the differential count as a percentage of the total nucleated cell count (preferred), or recorded as the number of nRBCs per 100 leukocytes.

4. Note any morphologic abnormalities of leukocytes.

5. Locate and evaluate any large or atypical cells you noted on scanning.

CLINICALLY IMPORTANT BLOOD FILM ABNORMALITIES
Erythrocytes

Erythrocyte morphology can be an important aid in the diagnosis of anemias, and sometimes in the diagnosis of other disorders. In general, regenerative anemias are associated with blood loss or hemolysis, whereas nonregenerative anemias suggest decreased erythropoiesis in the bone marrow. Keep in mind that several days are required for the regenerative response to become apparent in peripheral blood. Expected blood film findings in a regenerative anemia from any cause include increased polychromasia, nucleated red cells (typically metarubricytes), Howell-Jolly bodies, and occasionally basophilic stippling. Additional erythrocyte morphologic abnormalities together with other laboratory data and clinical findings can provide the clinician with important clues to the process underlying many regenerative anemias (Box 2).

The most common abnormalities that are readily detectable on blood films and are the most diagnostically useful are described below.

Polychromasia

Polychromatophils correspond to aggregate reticulocytes, which are identified with a vital stain such as new methylene blue (Fig. 3A). The reticulocyte count is a more sensitive measure of erythrocyte regeneration; all polychromatophils are reticulocytes, but not all reticulocytes can be appreciated as polychromatophils on a routine blood film. Nevertheless, identifying marked polychromasia on the blood film is a good indication of a regenerative response, and should trigger a confirmatory reticulocyte count. A strong regenerative response is usually seen with anemias caused by blood loss or hemolysis (after the marrow has had time to respond—usually 3 to 5 days). A strong regenerative response in a nonanemic or only slightly anemic animal is sometimes identified, and may be caused by some hereditary enzyme deficiencies (eg, PFK deficiency) or other causes of shortened red cell lifespan, or by hypoxia causing increased erythropoietin secretion [1]. Expect a slightly increased mean cell volume (MCV) and slightly decreased mean cell hemoglobin concentration (MCHC) when marked polychromasia is present. There are some species differences to keep in mind when evaluating polychromasia. Normal dogs may have up to 1% polychromatophils and cats up to 0.4% [2]. Dogs are capable of mounting a marked

Box 2: Regenerative anemia: differentiating hemolysis from blood loss

Suggestive of hemolysis

   Total protein normal

   Hemoglobinemia

   Hemoglobinuria

   Icterus

   Splenomegaly

   Heinz bodies or eccentrocytes (oxidative injury)

   Schistocytes and keratocytes (fragmentation injury due to microangiopathy, disseminated intravascular coagulation)

   Spherocytes ± agglutination, inflammatory leukogram (immune-mediated hemolytic anemia)

   Erythroparasites

Suggestive of blood loss

Acute

   Total protein decreased (both albumin and globulin)

   Mild thrombocytopenia (>100,000/μL, due to platelet loss with whole blood)

   Severe thrombocytopenia (<20,000/μL may cause hemorrhage)

   Acanthocytes and schistocytes (may be seen with hemangiosarcoma, which may cause bleeding)

   Schistocytes, keratocytes, and thrombocytopenia (seen with disseminated intravascular coagulation, which may cause bleeding)

Chronic

   Total protein normal or decreased

   Thrombocytosis

   Hypochromasia ± low MCV (iron deficiency)

   Keratocytes and schistocytes (iron deficiency)

regenerative response (>500,000 reticulocytes/μL), whereas 200,000/μL is considered a strong response in cats.

Hypochromasia

Hypochromasia refers to erythrocytes that are pale due to low hemoglobin content, and is recognized as increased central pallor (Fig. 3B). Iron deficiency is the most common cause of hypochromasia in dogs; other species' red cells usually do not appear hypochromic with iron deficiency. Red cells that are bowl-shaped (also called "punched-out") can mimic hypochromasia, but actually contain plenty of hemoglobin; these cells can be recognized by their thick rim of hemoglobin with an abrupt transition to the central clear area. If there

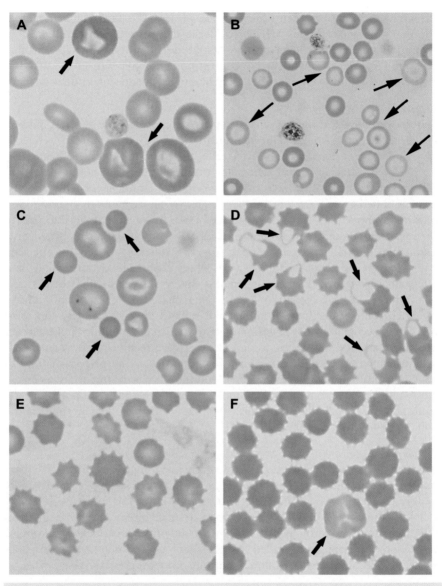

Fig. 3. (*A*) Polychromatophils (*arrows*) are larger than normal red cells and stain slightly basophilic. (*B*) Hypochromic red cells (*arrows*) in blood from an iron-deficient dog appear pale with a thin pale rim of hemoglobin. (*C*) Spherocytes (*arrows*) in blood from a dog with immune-mediated hemolytic anemia have no central pallor, appearing small and dense. (*D*) Keratocytes (*arrows*) are sometimes called "blister" cells or "helmet" cells. (*E*) Echinocytes with evenly spaced uniform projections. (*F*) Type 3 echinocytes from a dog with rattlesnake envenomation have very fine pointed projections. These appear to be spheroechinocytes. Note the polychromatophil (*arrow*) is not affected.

are large numbers of hypochromic red cells present, the mean cell hemoglobin concentration will be slightly decreased. Because the mean cell hemoglobin concentration is an average (hemoglobin ÷ hematocrit × 100), many hypochromic cells are required to lower the concentration; thus, hypochromasia may be evident on the slide even if the mean cell hemoglobin concentration is normal.

Spherocytes
Spherocytes have lost their normal biconcave shape and have become spheres, appearing slightly smaller and denser (darker red) than normal red cells (Fig. 3C). They are most easily detected in dogs because canine red cells normally have noticeable central pallor. They are extremely difficult to identify in cats and other species that have small red cells. In immune-mediated hemolytic anemia, spherocytes form when macrophages recognize antibody bound to red cells and remove part of the red cell membrane, causing the red cell to reform as a sphere. Presence of large numbers of spherocytes strongly suggests immune-mediated hemolytic anemia; however, spherocytes may also be seen with Heinz-body anemia, zinc toxicosis, and after a blood transfusion, and a few may be seen with microangiopathic injury due to vasculitis or disseminated intravascular coagulation [2]. Also note that spherocytes are not always present in animals that have immune-mediated hemolytic anemia. It takes some practice to recognize spherocytes, particularly when large numbers of them are present in a blood film (perhaps because there are relatively few normal cells with which to compare them). Thus, if spherocytes are suspected it is best to have a clinical pathologist review the blood film. It is very important to evaluate potential spherocytes in the monolayer of the blood film, as cells at the feathered edge are flattened and distorted, and often lose their normal central pallor, mimicking spherocytes.

Keratocytes
Keratocytes are formed from physical or chemical injury to red cells (which may occur secondary to iron deficiency, oxidative damage, or microangiopathic disease processes) (Fig. 3D). These cells are sometimes called "blister cells", because they may appear to have a small blister or vesicle in them that may rupture to form "helmet cells" with two projections. Cells with a single projection are sometimes called "apple-stem" cells. Keratocytes are more susceptible to intravascular trauma, and thus may progress to schistocytes.

Echinocytes
Echinocytes have numerous short, evenly spaced, uniform projections. They may be artifactual (due to slow-drying blood films, also known as "crenation"), but have also been associated with renal disease, electrolyte disorders, chemotherapy, lymphoma, and rattlesnake envenomation [2,3] (Fig. 3E). The echinocytes seen in dogs with rattlesnake envenomation are a special type, called type 3 echinocytes, which have large numbers of very fine pointed projections and affect all red cells except for polychromatophils; sometimes they form spheroechinocytes (spherocytes with the same very fine projections) (Fig. 3F). Type 3

echinocytes may be seen from 24 to 48 hours after envenomation, and are a reliable indicator of recent rattlesnake envenomation in suspect cases [3].

Schistocytes

Schistocytes are red cell fragments, resulting from shearing of red cells by intravascular trauma (Fig. 4A). This can occur during disseminated intravascular coagulation when fibrin strands are present in small vessels and physically cut the red cells; as a result red cells may lyse completely, seal the membrane resulting in fragmentation, or seal the membrane and reform as spherocytes. Schistocytes can also occur with hemangiosarcoma due to abnormal blood flow and localized disseminated intravascular coagulation; acanthocytes are often present in these animals as well [4]. Other processes with a microangiopathic component include vasculitis and heartworm disease. Schistocytes may be seen along with keratocytes in severe iron deficiency, and have also been reported in glomerulonephritis, liver disease, and heart failure [2].

Acanthocytes

In contrast to echinocytes, acanthocytes have a few blunt irregularly distributed spicules (Fig. 4B). They are thought to result from changes in the lipid content of red cell membranes, and thus have been associated with altered lipid metabolism as seen in liver disease, such as hepatic lipidosis [2]. However, they have also been associated with hemangiosarcoma in dogs, when they are frequently seen along with schistocytes [4,5].

Heinz bodies

Heinz bodies appear as small circular structures within or protruding from the red cell, and may be the same color as the cell or somewhat paler (Fig. 4C). They can be difficult to see on routine blood films, but stain dark blue with vital stains (ie, new methylene blue). Heinz bodies are denatured hemoglobin resulting from oxidative damage. Heinz bodies alter the cell membrane and make affected red cells more susceptible to both intra- and extravascular hemolysis. Feline red cells are especially susceptible to oxidative injury and Heinz body formation, and Heinz bodies may or may not be associated with hemolysis in cats. Heinz bodies have been associated with several systemic diseases in cats, including hyperthyroidism, lymphoma, and diabetes mellitus [6]. Specific oxidant toxins that have been associated with Heinz body formation in dogs and cats include onions, garlic, zinc, propylene glycol, and various drugs (acetaminophen, benzocaine, propofol, phenothiazine, Vitamin K, and others) [7–9]. Large numbers of Heinz bodies can cause an erroneously high hemoglobin value, which in turn may falsely increase the mean cell hemoglobin concentration.

Eccentrocytes

Eccentrocytes are the result of oxidative injury, and may be seen along with Heinz bodies in some cases (Fig. 4D). The cells have one edge of their membranes fused together and devoid of hemoglobin, so they appear dense on one side and clear on the other, with the edge of the membrane barely visible. The differentials are the same as for Heinz bodies.

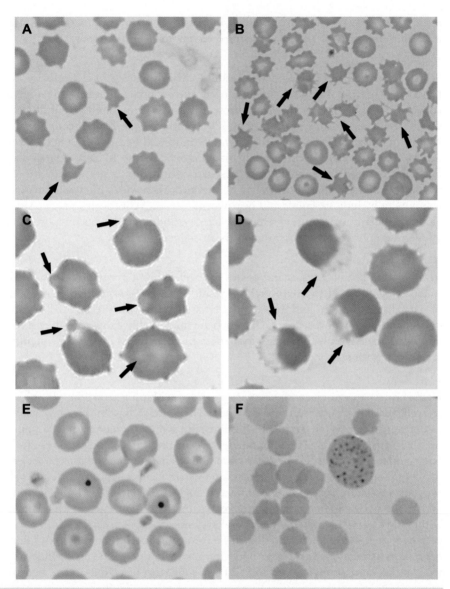

Fig. 4. (*A*) Schistocytes (*arrows*) are fragmented red cells associated with microangiopathic processes. (*B*) Acanthocytes (*arrows*) in blood from a dog that has splenic hemangiosarcoma have blunt irregularly spaced spicules. (*C*) Large Heinz bodies (*arrows*) in blood from an anemic cat suggest oxidative red cell injury. (*D*) Eccentrocytes (*arrows*) are also associated with oxidative damage. (*E*) Howell-Jolly bodies are round and basophilic, representing nuclear fragments. (*F*) Basophilic stippling (multiple small basophilic dots) can be seen with intensely regenerative anemia.

Howell-Jolly bodies
Howell-Jolly bodies are nuclear remnants, appearing as small round basophilic inclusions on a Wright's-stained blood film (Fig. 4E). They may be seen normally in small numbers, and increased numbers are associated with increased hematopoiesis (regenerative anemia) or splenic dysfunction. These should not be mistaken for hemoparasites.

Basophilic stippling
Basophilic stippling appears as numerous small basophilic dots inside red cells on a routine blood film, and reflects aggregated ribosomes in the cells (Fig. 4F). Basophilic stippling may be seen with intensely regenerative anemias in dogs and cats. Basophilic stippling (along with numerous nucleated red blood cells [nRBCs]) in the absence of a regenerative anemia suggests the possibility of lead poisoning.

Rouleaux
Red cells exhibit rouleaux formation when they "stack up" like a roll of coins (Fig. 5A). Some rouleaux formation is normal. Rouleaux is enhanced by increases in plasma proteins, particularly immunoglobulins and other inflammatory proteins. These proteins block the negative charges on red cell membranes, which normally allow red cells to repel one another. Rouleaux should not be confused with agglutination.

Agglutination
In contrast to rouleaux, agglutinating red cells adhere to each other in grape-like clusters due to antibody-mediated bridging between cells (Fig. 5B). When present, it indicates that red cells have been coated with antibody, and strongly suggests immune-mediated hemolytic anemia. It can be difficult to distinguish from rouleaux; a saline agglutination test should be performed to confirm agglutination when suspected. Marked agglutination may sometimes be seen grossly on the sides of the EDTA tube. Erythroparasites may be an underlying cause of agglutination, thus red cells should be examined carefully. Agglutination can cause multiple errors in hematology analyzer results (see later discussion).

Erythroparasites
Erythroparasites—parasites in or on red cells—may induce an immune-mediated hemolytic anemia, complete with agglutination and spherocytosis, and some may cause direct lysis of red cells (Fig. 5C–F). Parasites frequently recognized in cats include *Mycoplasma haemofelis* (previously *Hemobartonella felis*) and *Cytauxzoon felis* (in select areas of the country). *M haemofelis* is actually on, not in, red cells, and appears as small rod-shaped organisms on the red cell periphery or as ring-shaped structures on the cell. This organism will dissociate from red cells in vitro, and so freshly made blood smears are preferred for examination. In contrast, *C felis* is actually within red cells, and appears as small signet–ring-shaped piroplasms. The anemia associated with *C felis* is usually nonregenerative, which is unusual; most anemias associated with erythroparasites are

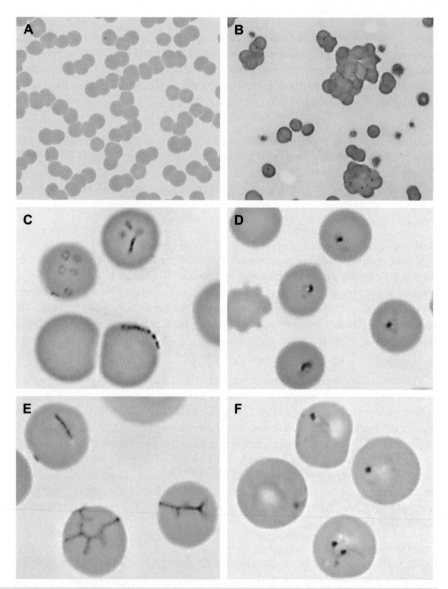

Fig. 5. (A) Rouleaux appears as "stacks of coins", and should not be confused with aggluti-nation. (B) Agglutination appears as "grape-like clusters", indicating antibody coated red cells. This image is from a cat that has immune-mediated hemolytic anemia secondary to *My-coplasma haemofelis* infection. (C) *Mycoplasma haemofelis* organisms in feline blood appear as basophilic rods, chains, and ring forms. (D) *Cytauxzoon felis* piroplasms in feline blood have an eccentric basophilic nucleus and small amount of clear cytoplasm. (E) *Mycoplasma haemocanis* organisms in canine blood frequently chain across the red cell. (F) *Babesia gibsoni* organisms in canine blood appear similar to *Cytauxzoon* piroplasms.

regenerative. Occasionally, large macrophages containing a schizont with developing *C felis* merozoites may be seen at the feathered edge of the blood film late in the course of the disease (Fig. 6A). Erythroparasites of dogs include *Mycoplasma haemocanis* (previously *Hemobartonella canis*), *Babesia gibsoni*, and *Babesia canis*. *M haemocanis* is of low pathogenicity, usually causing disease only in splenectomized or immunocompromised animals. It often appears as small chains of organisms across the surface of the red cell. *Babesia* organisms are a problem in select areas of the country. *B canis* forms large oval piroplasms, whereas *B gibsoni* looks much like *C felis*. *B gibsoni* has appeared in the United States more frequently since 1999, often in American Pit Bull and Staffordshire terriers [10,11].

Nucleated erythrocytes
Nucleated red blood cells, typically metarubricytes, may be present in peripheral blood for various reasons including: as part of a strongly regenerative bone marrow response to anemia, due to bone marrow injury allowing escape into circulation, splenectomy or splenic dysfunction, lead toxicity, and erythroid neoplasia (**Fig. 6B–E**). Erythroid neoplasia, typically in FeLV positive cats, can cause dramatic increases in nRBCs, often including more immature forms such as prorubricytes and rubriblasts. These cats may also have circulating megaloblasts exhibiting maturation dysynchrony (large nRBCs with an immature nucleus but hemoglobinized cytoplasm).

If present, nRBCs will be included in the "leukocyte" counts generated by most hematology analyzers and manual methods; these are really total nucleated cell counts, not leukocyte counts. When the nucleated cell count includes nRBCs, the simplest and most straightforward way to enumerate them is to include nRBCs in the differential count and generate an absolute number of nRBCs per μL by multiplying the percentage by the total cell count—the same as for neutrophils, lymphocytes, and other leukocytes. Historically, nRBCs have been left out of the differential count, instead reported as nRBC number per 100 leukocytes. In that case, the cell count must be corrected for the presence of the nRBCs before absolute numbers of leukocytes can be generated (nucleated cell count × 100 ÷ [100 + nRBCs] = corrected leukocyte count). This is less desirable for two reasons. First, it is an extra calculation step that is time consuming and introduces opportunity for error. Second, it is harder to interpret the number of nRBCs when they are reported as a relative number; 10 nRBCs per 100 leukocytes means something different when the leukocyte count is 100,000/μL versus 10,000/μL. If nRBCs are reported as the number per 100 leukocytes, you can calculate an absolute number of nRBCs using the following formula: corrected leukocyte count × (nRBC ÷ 100) = nRBC per μL.

Leukocytes
Leukocyte morphologic changes can provide key information important for complete blood cell count interpretation. For example, the total leukocyte count

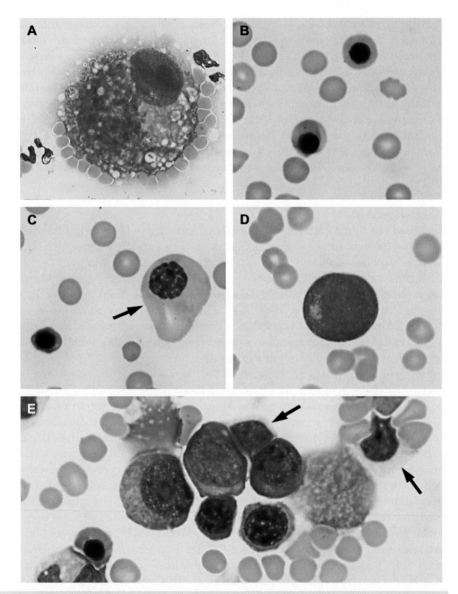

Fig. 6. (A) A large macrophage containing a *Cytauxzoon felis* schizont at the feathered edge of a blood film from a *C felis*-infected cat. Note the large nucleolus present in the macrophage's nucleus at the upper right; this is a typical finding. (B) Two metarubricytes from a cat that has a markedly regenerative anemia. (C) One metarubricyte and one megaloblast (*arrow*) from a cat that has FeLV-associated erythroid leukemia. The megaloblast is large with a relatively immature nucleus for its hemoglobinized cytoplasm (maturation dysynchrony). (D) A rubriblast from a cat that has erythroid leukemia. (E) All stages of immature erythroid cells in blood from a cat that has erythroid leukemia. Two normal lymphocytes are indicated by the arrows.

may be within normal limits, but if there is a marked left shift with toxic change a severe inflammatory process is present. Automated analyzers are not capable of quantifying a left shift, although the more sophisticated instruments can display cytograms that might suggest the presence of a left shift (these instruments are typically found in reference laboratories). Although hematology instruments claim 3-part or 5-part differentials, confirmation of the leukocyte distribution by visual evaluation of the blood film should be routine, with a manual differential preferred for any sick animal. Some of the important morphologic changes that should be recognized while examining the blood film at high power (100× oil objective) are listed below.

Immature neutrophils
Increased numbers of band neutrophils signifies a left shift, and defines an inflammatory leukogram (Fig. 7A). A severe left shift may result in metamyelocytes being released from the marrow, and sometimes even earlier precursors. The magnitude of the left shift is related to the severity of the underlying inflammation; a left shift with neutropenia or a degenerative left shift (immature forms outnumber segmented forms) is considered a poor prognostic sign if it is persistent.

Toxic change
Toxic changes in neutrophils include increased cytoplasmic basophilia, Döhle bodies, foamy vacuolation, toxic granulation (pink primary granules usually absent in mature cells), giant neutrophils, and "donut" neutrophils (nuclei are ring-shaped) (Fig. 7B). These changes reflect accelerated bone marrow production causing defective maturation, and are generally associated with severe inflammation, frequently due to sepsis. Usually there is a left shift present along with the toxic change. If the left shift is severe, toxic metamyelocytes may be difficult to differentiate from monocytes.

Pelger-Huet anomaly
Animals that have Pelger-Huet anomaly have an inability to segment the nuclei of all granulocytes (neutrophils, eosinophils, and basophils) (Fig. 7C). This is usually an inherited condition, although acquired forms have been reported. Granulocyte function is not affected. Although not common, it is important to recognize this condition so that it is not confused with a severe left shift. The key features are that the nuclei have the normal condensed chromatin associated with segmented neutrophils, and that all granulocytes are affected.

Reactive lymphocytes
Occasional reactive lymphocytes may be seen in blood films from animals undergoing antigenic stimulation (Fig. 7D). These cells may be larger than a neutrophil (in comparison to normal small lymphocytes, which are smaller than a neutrophil) with more abundant deep blue cytoplasm. Nuclei may be indented or convoluted, and the nuclear chromatin may appear normal (clumped and smudged) or immature (stippled). Nucleoli are generally not present. Reactive lymphocytes may be difficult to differentiate from neoplastic lymphocytes.

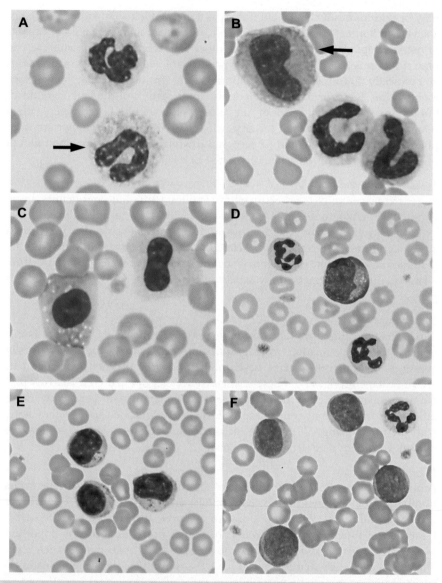

Fig. 7. (A) A band neutrophil (*arrow*) has a nonsegmented nucleus with parallel sides and less clumped chromatin than the segmented neutrophil above it. (B) A toxic neutrophil and band with basophilic, slightly vacuolated cytoplasm. Compare with the normal monocyte (*arrow*). (C) Pelger-Huet anomaly, an inability to segment nuclei, affects both neutrophils (*upper right*) and eosinophils (*lower left*). Note that the chromatin is mature and clumped. (D) A reactive lymphocyte that is larger than a neutrophil. Cytoplasm is deeply basophilic; the nuclear chromatin is immature. (E) Large granular lymphocytes (LGLs) have distinct azurophilic cytoplasmic granules. (F) Large atypical lymphocytes from a dog with lymphocytic leukemia. They are larger than the neutrophil, have immature chromatin and have indistinct nucleoli.

Large granular lymphocytes

Large granular lymphocytes have more abundant pale cytoplasm with discrete azurophilic (magenta) granules in the cytoplasm (Fig. 7E). Immunophenotyping has shown these cells are either CD8+ T-cells or NK cells [12]. Increased numbers are associated with Ehrlichial infections and chronic lymphocytic leukemia [13,14].

Atypical lymphocytes and lymphoblasts

Atypical lymphocytes and lymphoblasts are also larger than a neutrophil and contain nuclei with immature, stippled chromatin; lymphoblasts will also have distinct nucleoli (Fig. 7F). When present in large numbers these cells suggest acute lymphocytic leukemia or stage V lymphoma. However, they may be present in low numbers secondary to inflammatory disease. Lymphoblasts may appear morphologically identical to other leukemic blast cells such as myeloblasts.

Other neoplastic cells

Often, these are poorly differentiated hematopoietic cells that may or may not show morphologic evidence of their cell lineage (Fig. 8A). In acute leukemias, blast cells (containing nucleoli) of all lineages can have a similar appearance. A bone marrow evaluation is usually indicated, and additional tests such as cytochemical staining and immunophenotyping may be required. Chronic leukemias, in contrast, consist of well-differentiated leukocytes present in large numbers. Because large atypical cells and blast cells present significant diagnostic challenges, a fresh blood film should be sent to a clinical pathologist for consultation.

Inclusions

Microorganisms are occasionally seen within leukocytes, including *Ehrlichia* morula, *Hepatozoon* gamonts, *Histoplasma* organisms, and rarely bacteria (Fig. 8B–E). Abnormal cytoplasmic granules or vacuolation can be seen with lysosomal storage diseases (rare) and some leukemias. Consultation with a clinical pathologist is recommended whenever inclusions are suspected.

Mast cells

Mast cells are most frequently identified at the feathered edge of a blood film, and can be differentiated from basophils by their round nucleus and numerous dark granules that may obscure the nucleus (Fig. 8F). Mast cells may be seen in circulation in many inflammatory conditions as well as with mast cell neoplasia [15].

THE BLOOD FILM AS QUALITY CONTROL

Platelet Numbers

Platelet clumping can have a marked affect on the platelet count, whether generated by an automated analyzer, a manual hemocytometer count, or an estimate from the blood film. Therefore, before accepting any platelet count that is below normal, the blood film must be evaluated for the presence of clumps.

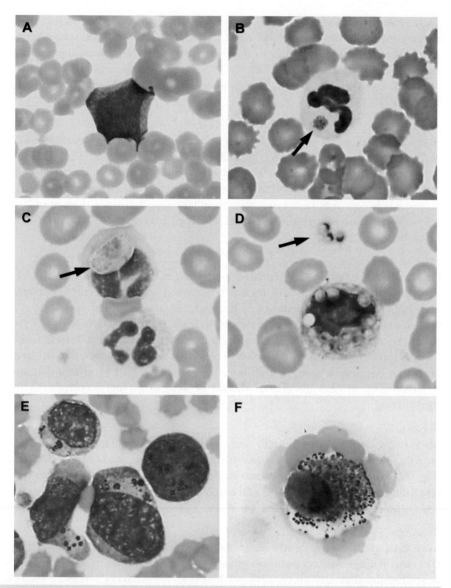

Fig. 8. (A) A blast cell (note the nucleolus) in blood from a dog that has myelogenous leukemia. Blast cells of all hematopoietic lineages can have a similar appearance. (B) An *Ehrlichia* morula in the neutrophil of a dog. (C) An *Hepatozoon* gamont within a canine leukocyte. (D) *Histoplasma* organisms free in the background (*arrow*) and phagocytized by a leukocyte in the blood from a dog with systemic histoplasmosis. (E) Large cytoplasmic granules within neoplastic lymphocytes in blood from a cat that has large granular lymphocytic (LGL) leukemia. (F) A mast cell at the feathered edge of a blood film from a dog with inflammatory disease.

Large clumps are usually evident at the feathered edge, but small clumps may also be observed in the monolayer or body of the film (Fig. 9A, B). Large clumps are usually not counted at all by the analyzer, whereas small clumps are sometimes counted as leukocytes (this occurs most often in feline samples.) Whenever clumps are noted, the generated platelet count or estimate should be interpreted as the minimum number of platelets present in the sample. If an accurate count is required, a new blood sample must be drawn.

Marked abnormalities often result if larger platelet clots are present in the sample (grossly visible clots). Such clots trap leukocytes, erythrocytes, and platelets, causing inaccurate cell counts. If the clots obstruct hematology instrument tubing, "short sampling" will occur, and none of the reported parameters will be correct. In addition, the hematology instrument will require cleaning

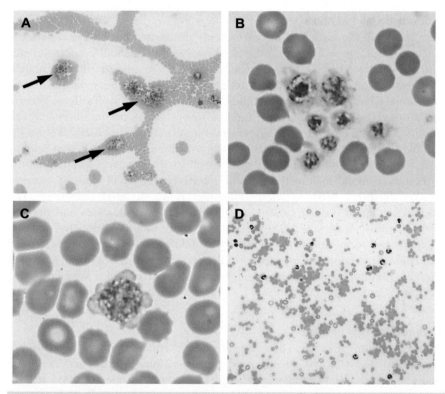

Fig. 9. (*A*) Small platelet clumps at the feathered edge (*arrows*) can be seen on low-power scanning, and will artifactually decrease the automated, manual, and estimated platelet counts. (*B*) A small platelet clump in the body of a blood film from a normal cat. Note that two platelets are larger than red cells. The large size and platelet clumping will artifactually decrease the platelet count. (*C*) A giant platelet in the blood of a thrombocytopenic dog suggests active thrombopoiesis. (*D*) Agglutination seen on low power (20× objective) in the body of a blood film from a dog that has immune-mediated hemolytic anemia.

before additional samples can be analyzed. Careful attention to the quality of the blood sample in the tube will prevent these kinds of problems.

Enlarged or giant platelets (larger than erythrocytes) usually indicate active thrombopoiesis, and in a thrombocytopenic animal suggest that decreased production in the marrow is not the cause of the thrombocytopenia (Fig. 9C) [16]. In normal cats, however, platelets are frequently close to the size of erythrocytes. This creates significant problems with automated platelet counts generated by impedance-based analyzers, which separate cells based on their size; large platelets will be counted as erythrocytes, artifactually lowering the platelet count. In addition, platelet clumping is frequent in feline blood samples. Because of these two problems, feline platelet counts are notoriously inaccurate. The platelet estimate from the blood film is often a better indication of the actual platelet count in cats, keeping in mind that platelet clumps will also affect the platelet estimate [17].

Nucleated Cell Numbers

Providing that the nucleated cells are evenly distributed on the blood film, the nucleated cell count from an automated analyzer or manual hemocytometer and the nucleated cell estimate from the blood film should roughly match. The main value of routinely performing an estimate is to verify the automated or manual count, and to prevent technical or instrument problems from becoming an ongoing source of error. Potential causes of inaccurate automated cell counts include sample quality issues (aged samples containing many lysed cells, samples that were not mixed well, samples containing clots that trap cells or plug instrument tubing), analyzer mechanical issues (incorrect sample volume aspiration, tubing malfunctions), and interferences (small platelet clumps, marked lipemia). Most of these difficulties result in falsely decreased cell counts, but small platelet clumps may be counted as leukocytes and marked lipemia rarely can cause falsely increased cell counts. Additionally, manual methods and most automated analyzers include nRBCs in the total nucleated cell count. It is important to recognize the presence of nRBCs when scanning the blood film; if more than a few metarubricytes are seen or if very immature erythroid precursors are present a manual differential should always be performed.

Erythrocyte Agglutination

Marked agglutination of erythrocytes is a fairly frequent finding in cases of immune-mediated hemolytic anemia, and can cause multiple errors in hematology analyzer results. Red cell aggregates may be counted as one large red cell, increasing the measured mean cell volume and decreasing the red blood cell count. Very large aggregates will not be counted at all, further decreasing the red blood cell count. Because the red blood cell count and mean cell volume are used by most analyzers to calculate the hematocrit, (hematocrit = mean cell volume × red blood cell count ÷ 10), agglutination can cause erroneous hematocrit values. In turn, the incorrect hematocrit can cause errors in the mean cell hemoglobin concentration, [mean cell hemoglobin concentration = (hemoglobin ÷ hematocrit) × 100]. Typically the mean cell hemoglobin concentration is falsely increased out of the reference interval. Generally a spun packed-cell volume will be more accurate in these cases, and should correspond to the measured hemoglobin; the hemoglobin should be about one third of the packed-cell volume.

Agglutination may be seen in the EDTA tube in severe cases, or suspected by evaluation of the blood film. On the blood film, agglutination is generally easiest to see in the body of the film while scanning at low power (using 10× or 20× objectives) (**Fig. 9D**). Suspected agglutination should be confirmed with a saline agglutination test. To perform this test, a drop of saline is applied to a clean slide and an applicator stick is used to pick up a tiny amount of blood from the EDTA tube and mix it gently into the saline. A coverslip is applied, and the preparation evaluated on the microscope using the 10× or 20× objectives. The condenser should be lowered to provide adequate contrast because the preparation is unstained. True agglutination will remain, whereas rouleaux will disperse in saline.

SUMMARY

Blood film evaluation remains one of the most diagnostically important parts of the complete blood count, and must not be overlooked when in-clinic analyses are performed with automated hematology instruments. The value of the blood film for routine quality control cannot be overemphasized. Because in-clinic hematology analyses are typically performed by veterinary technicians, veterinarians are encouraged to find technicians with a particular interest in laboratory work and promote that interest with appropriate continuing education in hematology. If in-clinic blood film review by a competent individual is not possible, or if unusual or confusing abnormalities are observed, freshly made blood films should be sent to a veterinary clinical pathologist for evaluation.

References

[1] Harvey JW. Pathogenesis, laboratory diagnosis, and clinical implications of erythrocyte enzyme deficiencies in dogs, cats, and horses. Vet Clin Pathol 2006;35(2):144–56.

[2] Tvedten H, Weiss DJ. Classification and laboratory evaluation of anemia. In: Feldman EC, Zinkl JG, Jain NC, editors. Schalm's veterinary hematology. 5th edition. Philadelphia: Lippincott Williams & Wilkins; 2000. p. 143–50.

[3] Brown DE, Meyer DJ, Wingfield WE, et al. Echinocytosis associated with rattlesnake envenomation in dogs. Vet Pathol 1994;31(6):654–7.

[4] Ng CY, Mills JN. Clinical and haematological features of haemangiosarcoma in dogs. Aust Vet J 1985;62(1):1–4.

[5] Weiss DJ, Kristensen A, Papenfuss N. Qualitative evaluation of irregularly spiculated red blood cells in the dog. Vet Clin Pathol 1993;22(4):117–21.

[6] Christopher MM. Relation of endogenous Heinz bodies to disease and anemia in cats: 120 cases (1978–1987). J Am Vet Med Assoc 1989;194(8):1089–95.

[7] Andress JL, Day TK, Day D. The effects of consecutive day propofol anesthesia on feline red blood cells. Vet Surg 1995;24(3):277–82.

[8] Lee KW, Yamato O, Tajima M, et al. Hematologic changes associated with the appearance of eccentrocytes after intragastric administration of garlic extract to dogs. Am J Vet Res 2000;61(11):1446–50.

[9] Stockham SL, Scott MA. Fundamentals of veterinary clinical pathology. Ames (IA): Iowa State Press; 2002. p. 130–1.

[10] Birkenheuer AJ, Levy MG, Savary KC, et al. Babesia gibsoni infections in dogs from North Carolina. J Am Anim Hosp Assoc 1999;35(2):125–8.

[11] Macintire DK, Boudreaux MK, West GD, et al. Babesia gibsoni infection among dogs in the southeastern United States. J Am Vet Med Assoc 2002;220(3):325–9.

[12] McDonough SP, Moore PF. Clinical, hematologic, and immunophenotypic characterization of canine large granular lymphocytosis. Vet Pathol 2000;37(6):637–46.

[13] Weiser MG, Thrall MA, Fulton R, et al. Granular lymphocytosis and hyperproteinemia in dogs with chronic ehrlichiosis. J Am Anim Hosp Assoc. 1991;27:84–8.

[14] Vernau W, Moore PF. An immunophenotypic study of canine leukemias and preliminary assessment of clonality by polymerase chain reaction. Vet Immunol Immunopathol 1999;69(2–4):145–64.

[15] McManus PM. Frequency and severity of mastocytemia in dogs with and without mast cell tumors: 120 cases (1995–1997). J Am Vet Med Assoc 1999;215(3):355–7.

[16] Russell KE, Grindem CB. Secondary thrombocytopenia. In: Feldman EC, Zinkl JG, Jain NC, editors. Schalm's veterinary hematology. 5th edition. Philadelphia: Lippincott Williams & Wilkins; 2000. p. 487–95.

[17] Norman EJ, Barron RC, Nash AS, et al. Prevalence of low automated platelet counts in cats: comparison with prevalence of thrombocytopenia based on blood smear estimation. Vet Clin Pathol 2001;30(3):137–40.

Vet Clin Small Anim 37 (2007) 267–282

VETERINARY CLINICS
SMALL ANIMAL PRACTICE

Determining the Significance of Persistent Lymphocytosis

Anne C. Avery, VMD, PhD[a,b,*], Paul R. Avery, VMD, PhD[b]

[a]Clinical Immunopathology Service, 300 West Drake Street, College of Veterinary Medicine and Biomedical Sciences, Colorado State University, Fort Collins, CO 80523, USA
[b]Department of Microbiology, Immunology, and Pathology, College of Veterinary and Biomedical Sciences, Campus Delivery 1619, Colorado State University, Fort Collins, CO 80523, USA

W hen a small animal patient presents with repeatable lymphocytosis, the differential list suggested by clinicians and clinical pathologists usually includes antigenic stimulation from infectious disease, antigenic stimulation, or lymphocyte activation from autoimmune disease, hypoadrenocorticism, thymoma, and lymphoproliferative disorders. In rare cases, congenital immunodeficiency disorders might also be considered. When the lymphocytes are described as small and mature or reactive and clinical signs and other laboratory changes are nonspecific, the clinician is faced with a diagnostic dilemma: is this a neoplastic process (chronic lymphocytic leukemia [CLL] or lymphoma) or a nonneoplastic reactive process? Here, the authors have tried to create a narrower and more informative differential list for such patients. They have specifically not included excitement-induced lymphocytosis because this would be considered a transient and generally not repeatable cause of lymphocytosis. The focus in this review is on the primary literature, together with emerging data from the Clinical Immunopathology Service at Colorado State University.

First, the authors provide a review of current knowledge of lymphocytosis in nonneoplastic conditions. They conclude that the list of major differentials for persistent nonneoplastic lymphocyte expansion in dogs and cats is short and that most of these conditions are relatively uncommon. Persistent lymphocytosis of small, mature, or reactive lymphocytes is most commonly the result of CLL or lymphoma. The first step in distinguishing nonneoplastic from neoplastic lymphocytosis is immunophenotyping by flow cytometry to determine the phenotypic diversity of the circulating cells. Clonality testing using the polymerase chain reaction [PCR] for antigen receptor rearrangements (PARR) assay is a useful second step in cases in which the phenotype data are equivocal.

*Corresponding author. Department of Microbiology, Immunology, and Pathology, College of Veterinary and Biomedical Sciences, Campus Delivery 1619, Colorado State University, Fort Collins, CO 80523. E-mail address: anne.avery@colostate.edu (A.C. Avery).

0195-5616/07/$ – see front matter
doi:10.1016/j.cvsm.2006.11.001

Once the diagnosis of malignancy has been established, the immunophenotype also provides prognostic information in dogs.

LYMPHOCYTOSIS IN NONNEOPLASTIC CONDITIONS
Canine Infectious Disease

Chronic infectious disease is often listed as a differential for lymphocytosis in dogs. Although studies that systematically analyze lymphocytosis as a primary presenting complaint are lacking, a review of the literature suggests that with the exception of *Ehrlichia canis* infection, lymphocytosis is not a common feature of canine chronic infectious disease. In reviewing these studies, the authors assumed that if hematologic abnormalities (eg, neutrophilia) were noted, the lack of comment on lymphocytosis meant that the lymphocyte counts were not elevated. Lymphocytosis has not been reported in case series for several protozoal infections. These diseases include *Trypanosoma cruzi* [1,2], *Babesia gibsoni* [3,4], *Babesia canis* [5] infections; hepatozoonosis [6]; and experimental infection with *Leishmania infantum* [7]. Lymphocytosis was reported in 8 of 23 foxhounds naturally infected with *L infantum* (the highest value was 15,000 cells/µL), but some of these dogs also had serologic evidence of *E canis* infection [8]. The nematode infection *Spirocerca lupi* was associated with lymphocytosis as high as 8000 cells/µL (8 of 32 cases [9]). *Dirofilaria immitis* was associated with a high lymphocyte percentage, but absolute counts were not reported [10].

The chronic bacterial infections that cause Lyme disease and Rocky Mountain spotted fever do not seem to be associated with lymphocytosis. The authors could find no reports describing lymphocytosis associated with naturally occurring or experimental disease. Although monocytosis was found in 4 of 5 dogs with Rocky Mountain spotted fever [11], no dogs were reported to have lymphocytosis, and lymphocytosis was also not reported in experimental Rocky Mountain spotted fever infection [12]. Naturally occurring granulocytic ehrlichiosis in 14 dogs was not associated with lymphocytosis [13], but granulocytic ehrlichial infection in the experimental setting was associated with mild lymphocytosis (4500 cells/µL) during the recovery phase [14]. These lymphocytes were characterized as being blasts, with some characterized as having granules.

By contrast, lymphocytosis is a notable feature of chronic *E canis* infection. Numerous studies have shown that naturally occurring *E canis* infection can result in lymphocytosis with values up to 17,000 lymphocytes/µL [15–19], although not all case series describe lymphocytosis [20]. Anecdotal reports and the experience of some clinicians and clinical pathologists suggest that lymphocyte counts up to 30,000 cells/µL are possible in *E canis* infection. The lymphocyte response consists of cells with a large granular lymphocyte (LGL) phenotype [16,17,21], which were shown to be CD8+ T cells. Experimental *E canis* infection does not seem to have the same effect on lymphocyte count, but mild CD8+ T-cell expansion has been found [22]. Therefore, an important differential for lymphocytosis in dogs is *E canis* infection, and the frequency with which lymphocytosis is associated with *E canis* seems to be unique to this disease.

Feline Infectious Disease

There is less information about the development of lymphocytosis in feline infectious disease. It was not described in association with *Cytauxzoon felis* (34 cases [23]), natural *Toxoplasma gondii* infection (2 cases [24]), natural *Anaplasma phagocytophilum* infection (5 cases [25]), feline heartworm infection (50 cases [26]), or experimental *Mycoplasma felis* infection (18 cats [27]). Experimental *T gondii* infection did result in mild lymphocytosis (9000 cells/µL [28]), and 3 of 21 cases of naturally acquired *M felis* developed lymphocytosis with counts between 7000 and 9000 cells/µL [29]. Three cats infected with an *E canis*–like organism developed anemia, thrombocytopenia and, in 1 case, pancytopenia similar to the canine infection, but none had lymphocytosis [30]. There are reports of feline immunodeficiency virus (FIV)–associated lymphocytosis (1 of 5 cats with a lymphocyte count of 13,000 cells/µL [31]), and lymphocytosis was present in 8 of 46 FIV-positive cats in a study by Hopper and colleagues [32]. At least 2 of the cats in this series had a lymphoid malignancy, and given the known association between FIV and B-cell lymphoma, it is important to establish that cases of lymphocytosis in FIV infection are not the result of malignancy. It is important to note that in a large study of 30 cats experimentally infected with several different FIV isolates and followed for 15 years, no cat developed lymphocytosis at any time during the study (Mathiason C and Hoover E, unpublished data, 1999). Taken together, the available primary literature indicates that mild lymphocytosis can occasionally be associated with several feline infectious diseases, but this finding is uncommon.

Autoimmune Disease

A finding of lymphocytosis in cases of canine autoimmune disease also seems to be rare. Immune-mediated hemolytic anemia (IMHA) is probably the best-studied canine autoimmune disease, yet lymphocytosis was not reported in any study series [33–35]. In contrast, however, two reports that examined presumptive cases of IMHA in a total of 22 cats found that 9 had lymphocytosis, with one case as high as 20,000 cells/µL [36,37]. Lymphocytosis was not reported in other canine systemic autoimmune diseases, and presumptive autoimmune diseases include systemic lupus erythematosus (in which lymphopenia was a dominant feature [38]), rheumatoid arthritis, and nonseptic and nonerosive polyarthritis [39].

Other Causes

Lymphocytosis has been associated with hypoadrenocorticism in dogs and cats. Studies vary on the incidence of lymphocytosis in dogs with Addison's disease, ranging from 5% to 10% of patients, with the highest lymphocyte count recorded being 13,000 cells/µL [40–42], although in a report focusing on patients with glucocorticoid deficiency only, no cases of lymphocytosis were found [43]. Cats with hypoadrenocorticism can also present with lymphocytosis (20% of cases in the single case series that has been reported [44]). Therefore, although only a few animals with Addison's disease have lymphocytosis, it should be considered a differential for unexplained mild persistent lymphocytosis.

Another endocrine disease that can be associated with lymphocytosis in cats is hyperthyroidism. In a comprehensive study of clinical data from cats with hyperthyroidism, Thoday and Mooney [45] found that 7% of 57 cats studied had lymphocytosis, with the highest lymphocyte count being 9000 cells/μL. Treatment of hyperthyroidism with methimazole can also cause lymphocytosis [46].

Thymomas in people have occasionally been associated with lymphocytosis consisting of CD4 and CD8+ T cells [47]. These cells are likely present because of increased production of nonneoplastic T cells, whose growth and differentiation are stimulated by the neoplastic thymic epithelium. Thymomas in dogs and cats can also present with concurrent lymphocytosis, although this is not described in all case series [48]. Of two cases reported in one study [49], one dog had a lymphocyte count of 19,000 cells/μL and the lymphocyte count of the other dog was within normal limits. The authors have evaluated nine cases of canine thymoma through the Clinical Immunopathology Service at Colorado State University (five of these are reported in the article by Lana and colleagues [50]) for the purpose of immunophenotyping aspirates from the tumor. In the complete blood cell counts (CBCs) available from these nine cases, two dogs had lymphocytosis. One cat with thymoma and lymphocytosis was reported in the article by Weiss [37], and a single cat had a high lymphocyte count (7000 cell/μL). Thus, thymoma should be included as a differential for lymphocytosis, although it is seen in only a few cases.

Postvaccination lymphocytosis is listed as a differential for an increased lymphocyte count in some references. The literature does not support this as a routine finding. In a study of 92 mixed-breed dogs, four commercially available polyvalent vaccines caused an actual decrease in circulating lymphocytes on days 3, 5 and 7 after vaccination [51]. Miyamoto and colleagues [52] demonstrated a similar decrease in lymphocyte count in puppies and adult dogs at day 7 after vaccination. A study examining the response of racing Greyhounds to a traditional or intense vaccination schedule failed to demonstrate any increase in circulating lymphocytes in samples taken biweekly during the 6-month study [53].

Summary of Nonneoplastic Lymphocytosis

Overall, review of the literature suggests that when presented with a case of persistent lymphocytosis, there is a relatively small list of nonneoplastic conditions to consider. In terms of infectious disease, *E canis* infection in dogs can result in significant lymphocytosis. Increased lymphocyte counts have been reported in canine *S lupi* and *L infantum* infections. Some reports of cats infected with *T gondii* and *M felis* have documented lymphocytosis, and a subset of cats with FIV infection may have lymphocytosis, but an underlying malignancy would also be a consideration in this disease. Lymphocytosis has been reported in some cats with IMHA, but this has not been reported in dogs. In a few cases, metabolic diseases, such as hypoadrenocorticism and feline hyperthyroidism, have been associated with persistent lymphocytosis. Finally, thymoma has been associated with benign expansion of peripheral lymphocytes in a small number of feline and canine cases.

NEOPLASTIC LYMPHOCYTOSIS

Lymphoproliferative disorders often present with peripheral lymphocytosis. CLL, acute lymphoblastic leukemia (ALL), and lymphoma with circulating neoplastic cells (stage V lymphoma) are the three forms of lymphoid malignancy in which lymphocytosis is a primary feature.

Chronic Lymphocytic Leukemia

CLL in people and animals involves the transformation and expansion of mature-appearing lymphocytes. The diagnosis of CLL in people requires lymphocytosis of greater than 5000 cells/µL of mature-appearing lymphocytes that express specific surface markers. CLL in people is primarily an expansion of immunophenotypically atypical B lymphocytes, and the disease usually has a prolonged clinical course. In people, it is thought that these cells arise from the bone marrow.

In veterinary medicine, there is no consensus on the criteria for making the diagnosis of CLL, partly because the immunophenotype of the cells is usually normal and B- and T-cell forms occur. Furthermore, it is likely that one or more subtypes of CLL arise in the spleen rather than in the bone marrow [21], making marrow involvement potentially unhelpful in establishing a diagnosis. Canine and feline CLL patients are often asymptomatic at presentation, with lymphocytosis ranging from 6000 to greater than 200,000 cells/µL [54,55]. Peripheral cytopenias tend to occur in a relatively small subset of cases and are generally mild (reviewed in the article by Workman and Vernau [56]). Canine CLL has been described as an indolent disease, although survival times can vary greatly [55]. Less is known about survival in feline CLL. Workman and colleagues [57] presented survival data for 17 cats with CLL and showed that treated cats (8 of 17 cats) had a mean survival of 28 months, whereas untreated cats (which were generally not treated because they tended to have severe disease and a poorer prognosis) survived 1 to 6 months.

Lymphoma

Lymphoma can also present as lymphocytosis. Published studies have reported a range of estimates of lymphocytosis associated with canine lymphoma of 7% [58], 28% [59], 37% [60], and 65% [61]. Fewer studies are available for cats; in one report, 5% of 97 cats with lymphoma had absolute lymphocytosis, with values reaching 80,000 cells/µL [62].

It is not clear whether some cases of lymphoma with lymphocytosis might be considered primary leukemia with lymph node involvement. In people, the nomenclature of human small lymphocytic lymphoma and leukemia has evolved to reflect the observation that lymph node infiltration is not uncommon in human CLL. Therefore, CLL and small B-cell lymphoma are considered together as one disease entity (CLL/small lymphocytic lymphoma). As discussed elsewhere in this article, this grouping of two disease entities might be appropriate in canine CLL as well.

Acute Lymphoblastic Leukemia

ALL is a rapidly fatal disease [54] that generally does not pose a diagnostic dilemma. Typical canine ALL presents with large numbers of circulating lymphoblasts and commonly has coexisting peripheral cytopenias. Therefore, malignancy can often be diagnosed by morphology alone, although immunophenotyping may help to assign a lineage in cases in which morphology cannot determine if the leukemia is lymphoid or myeloid.

Distinguishing Reactive from Neoplastic Expansions

In the previous sections, the authors outlined the nonneoplastic and neoplastic causes of lymphocytosis in small animal patients. When presented with a patient with persistent lymphocytosis, the first decision a clinician must make is whether the lymphocytosis is neoplastic or not. Such a distinction can be difficult when using clinical signs and lymphocyte morphology alone. Clinical signs in many of the diseases described may be nonspecific, and lymphocyte morphology may reveal only small, mature, or reactive lymphocytes. Lymphocyte morphology has been shown to be of limited use in distinguishing cell phenotype in veterinary and human medicine [54,63].

Several assays can be used to aid in the distinction between reactive and neoplastic lymphocyte populations (reviewed in the article by Avery and Avery [64]): (1) demonstrating a phenotypically homogeneous expanded lymphocyte population with or without the presence of aberrant antigen expression, (2) establishing cellular clonality, (3) identifying chromosomal abnormalities, and (4) identifying the presence of an oncogene associated with the malignancy. The first two methods are now readily available in veterinary medicine. The latter two are less well developed; however, the full sequence of the canine genome [65,66] and work by Breen and colleagues [67] to develop molecular methods of examining chromosomal aberrations should facilitate the development of future diagnostic assays. For the remainder of this review, the authors discuss methods that are now routinely available to practitioners: immunophenotyping and clonality assessment.

Immunophenotyping Using Flow Cytometry

Flow cytometry is the method of choice for immunophenotypic analysis. The methodology has been thoroughly reviewed in a previous issue in this series [56]. The value of flow cytometry lies in its ability to detect the expression of multiple antigens on the surface of lymphocytes efficiently. A continually expanding number of species-specific and cross-reactive antibodies for labeling canine and feline hematopoietic cells makes more detailed multiparameter flow cytometry possible [54,68]. Commercially available directly conjugated antibodies recognizing canine CD3 and CD5 (all T cells), CD4 (T-cell subset), CD8 (T-cell subset), CD21 (B cells), CD34 (precursor cells), and CD45 (a panleukocyte antigen) are all useful to characterize circulating lymphocytes. The commercially available repertoire of antibodies for feline immunophenotyping is more limited.

Lymphocytosis caused by leukemia or lymphoma is characterized by homogeneous expansion of cells with a single phenotype, whereas reactive lymphocyte expansions are likely to be heterogeneous, involving multiple lymphocyte subsets. Thus, the first immunophenotypic criterion suggesting malignancy is homogeneous expansion of lymphocytes, such as CD21+ cells (B cells) or CD8+ cells (T-cell subset). An important exception to this concept is the homogeneous expansion of CD8+ T cells in *E canis* infection. The authors know of no other disease in dogs or cats that causes a similar homogeneous reactive lymphocyte expansion.

Immunophenotyping by flow cytometry is a service that is now being provided by an increasing number of laboratories, most of which are in veterinary schools. There is no consensus as to the best combination of antibodies, the methods of cell preparation, how results are reported, or cost. Because of this diversity, it is probably best to find one laboratory and to use that service consistently so that the clinician can build familiarity with the interpretation of results.

Immunophenotype of Canine Chronic Lymphocytic Leukemia

Canine CLL is primarily a CD8+ T-cell disease. Vernau and Moore [54] examined 73 cases of canine CLL and determined that 73% were of T-cell origin, whereas only 26% expressed B-cell markers. Most T-cell leukemias were of the CD8+ subset, and many of these had an LGL morphology. Similarly, Ruslander and colleagues [69] found that 68% of canine CLLs were CD8+. A smaller subset of CLLs are composed of B cells (CD21+), and CD4+ T-cell CLLs seem to be rare. Immunophenotyping of CLLs by the authors' laboratory produced similar results [70].

Immunophenotype of Feline Chronic Lymphocytic Leukemia

There is little information about feline CLL in the literature. Workman and colleagues [57] presented a series of 20 cases of feline CLL whose lymphocyte counts ranged from 22,000 to 575,000 cells/μL. In that series, the predominant phenotype was CD4+ T cell. The authors' laboratory has phenotyped 60 cases of homogeneous lymphocyte expansion in cats with lymphocyte counts greater than 8000 cells/μL. Forty-two percent of these were CD4+; these cases had lymphocyte counts that ranged from 8000 to 125,000 cells/μL. Eleven percent of the 60 cases had homogeneous expansion of B cells (as determined by the expression of CD21). These cases tended to have a lower lymphocyte count, with the highest being 37,000 cells/μL. The remainder were a mixture of CD8+, CD4+8+, CD4−CD8−CD5+, and null cell. The authors do not have survival data for these cats yet; however, such studies are clearly a high priority to aid veterinarians and owners in making informed choices. A broader range of antibodies for feline studies is also an important goal.

Aberrant Antigen Expression

Aberrant antigen expression can further support the diagnosis of malignancy [71,72], because reactive lymphocytes retain expression of their normal constellation of antigens. Human T-cell leukemias are characterized by their tendency to lose expression of normal T-cell antigens or to express aberrant combinations of antigens [73]. In one study of 87 human malignant T-cell disorders, Gorczyca and colleagues [74] found that complete loss of any T-cell antigen (CD2, CD5, or CD7) or the panleukocyte antigen CD45 was diagnostic for malignancy. Aberrant antigen expression (failure to express CD4 or CD8 or coexpression of these two markers) was reported by Vernau and Moore [54] on 10 of 73 canine cases of CLL. Nevertheless, one of the drawbacks of older studies is that directly conjugated antibodies, which facilitate multicolor fluorescence, were not available, making aberrant antigen expression difficult to detect. In the authors' experience, almost half of T-cell leukemias (11 of 26 cases) during a 1-year period exhibited aberrant antigen expression (no expression of CD4 or CD8, loss of the panleukocyte antigen CD45, and occasional loss of the T-cell antigen CD5). Loss of expression of CD4 and CD8 or loss of CD5 expression has been associated with more rapid disease progression in human cases of adult T-cell leukemia [75]. Precursor T-cell ALL that lacks CD5 or CD4 expression has an increased risk of treatment failure and shorter event-free survival [76,77]. The authors' analysis of 89 cases of canine leukemia has not shown any significant survival difference in dogs with T-cell leukemias that lack CD4 and CD8 or CD45 expression as compared with phenotypically normal T-cell leukemias [78]. Thus, although aberrant antigen expression can be used to help make the diagnosis of neoplastic lymphocytosis, the more common variants do not seem to have prognostic significance in dogs. Too few cases of feline leukemia with aberrant antigen expression have been documented to reach similar conclusions in cats.

Determination of Lymphocyte Clonality

In cases in which the lymphocyte count is not markedly elevated and the lymphocytes do not exhibit aberrant antigen expression, additional support for the diagnosis of malignancy can be obtained from clonality testing by the PARR assay [79]. In human medicine, determination of clonality by detecting rearranged antigen receptor genes is the test of choice if routine cytology, histology, and immunophenotyping are not able to provide a definitive diagnosis of malignancy [80]. The principle behind this assay has been described by Avery and Avery [64] and Workman and Vernau [56]. Briefly, DNA is extracted from lymphocytes, and the size of the antigen receptor hypervariable region is determined by PCR. In B cells, the antigen receptor is immunoglobulin, and in T cells, it is the T-cell receptor. Because the size of the hypervariable region differs slightly in each lymphocyte, the finding of a single-sized hypervariable region indicates that all the lymphocytes are derived from a single clone and are most likely neoplastic. Reactive lymphocytes are derived from multiple different clones. Thus, the finding of a clonal population of lymphocytes by means of the PARR assay, coupled with homogeneous expansion of lymphocytes based on immunophenotyping, is strong evidence of neoplasia. To date, the authors know of only a single exception to this theory. *E canis* infection in dogs can cause not only homogeneous expansion of CD8 T cells but, in rare cases, clonal expansion [54,79]. Thus, in dogs positive for *E canis*, the response to treatment for *E canis* infection may be the best diagnostic tool for determining if lymphocytosis is attributable to infection or to an underlying malignancy.

Clonality testing in dogs and cats is presently established at two institutions (Colorado State University and the University of California, Davis), but it is likely that it will be available through other laboratories in the future. It is important that as laboratories develop this assay, they provide sensitivity and specificity numbers for their assay; published results from one laboratory do not translate to another because of the wide variation in the way the assay is performed. The sensitivity of the Colorado State University assay in dogs is 80%, and the specificity is 92%, but other laboratories may have different results. The authors estimate that the primers used in their laboratory at the present time can detect approximately 60% of confirmed feline lymphomas and leukemias, and they are working toward developing better reagents for cats.

Phenotypic homogeneity, aberrant antigen expression, and clonality can together distinguish reactive from neoplastic lymphocytosis. Immunophenotyping by flow cytometry is valuable not only for establishing a diagnosis but for predicting prognosis in cases of canine neoplastic lymphocytosis. In the following section, the authors summarize data from their study of a series of dogs with neoplastic lymphocytosis in which they correlated immunophenotype and other parameters with outcome.

Immunophenotyping Predicts Prognosis in Canine Lymphocytosis

Peripheral blood from 208 dogs with lymphocytosis was submitted to the Clinical Immunology Service at Colorado State University for immunophenotyping. A total of 202 of the 208 cases had homogeneous expansion (>80% of the lymphocytes) of one lymphocyte phenotype or aberrant antigen expression. Of these, clinical information and follow-up data were available for 89 cases. Thirty-one percent of these dogs had homogeneous expansion of B cells, 24% had homogeneous expansion of CD8+ T cells, 20% had expansion of CD34+ progenitor cells, 14% had CD5+ T cells that lacked CD4 or CD8 expression, 6% expressed other aberrant antigens, and 5% had homogeneous expansion of CD4+ T cells. The authors chose the B-cell and CD8+ T-cell groups for further analysis. They purposely included all cases with homogeneous expansion of circulating lymphocytes, knowing that the cases would encompass stage V lymphomas and primary leukemias. The authors are commonly asked to distinguish between these two entities; however, specific phenotypic markers to make this distinction are lacking. They were hopeful that more objective prognostic indicators would emerge to help distinguish between neoplastic T-cell and B-cell expansions as well as within phenotypes.

Canine B-Cell Lymphocytosis: Cell Size Matters

The distinction between human CLL/small lymphocytic lymphoma and other B-cell lymphomas with circulating atypical cells is made primarily based on cellular phenotype, because CLL/small lymphocytic lymphoma consists of B cells that express the T-cell marker CD5 [81]. Canine B-cell leukemia does not express CD5 [54] and is immunophenotypically indistinguishable from canine B-cell lymphoma (the most common form [82,83]) using commercially available antibodies. Therefore, the authors examined all cases of B-cell lymphocytosis, as defined by greater than 5000 lymphocytes/μL and greater than 80% CD21+ cells, and segregated them by size [78]. Dogs whose circulating lymphocytes were large (presumed stage V lymphoma or prolymphocytic/lymphoblastic leukemia) had a significantly shorter median survival time (115 days) than those with small circulating lymphocytes (CLL/small lymphocytic lymphoma, median survival not reached; $P = .035$). In the authors' cases series, all the dogs with circulating small CD21+ lymphocytes had corroborating evidence of neoplastic transformation, including (1) a lymphocyte count greater than 30,000 cells/μL or (2) cytologic evidence supporting a diagnosis of leukemia or lymphoma in bone marrow or lymph nodes. It is important to note that more than half of the dogs with circulating, small, mature-appearing CD21+ lymphocytes had detectable peripheral lymphadenopathy, suggesting that the designation of small lymphocytic lymphoma/CLL may be appropriate in dogs as well.

Canine T-Cell Lymphocytosis: Cell Numbers Matters

The two most commonly used clinical staging systems to predict prognosis in human B-cell CLL do not take into account initial lymphocyte count [84], and when initial lymphocyte counts have been specifically studied, they have not provided prognostic information [85]. The authors have found this to be true in dogs with small cell B-cell leukemias as well. When the more common CD8+ T-cell variant of canine CLL was examined, however, the initial lymphocyte count had a significant impact on survival. Dogs that presented with fewer than 30,000 lymphocytes/μL had a median survival time of 1098 days (indolent form), whereas those dogs with an initial lymphocyte count greater than 30,000 lymphocytes/μL had a median survival time of 131 days (aggressive form; $P < .008$) [78]. The dogs with fewer than 30,000 CD8+ lymphocytes/μL had additional evidence supporting a diagnosis of neoplasia, including (1) PCR positivity for a clonal T-cell receptor rearrangement, (2) aberrant antigen expression (loss of CD45), (3) atypical appearance of the circulating lymphocytes, or (4) persistence of the lymphocytosis with negative serology for *E canis*. Because longitudinal data were not available for most cases, the authors could not determine if indolent and aggressive forms represent ends of a single disease spectrum or if they are two discrete entities. As described previously, the authors also found that cases of canine neoplastic lymphocytosis with aberrant antigen expression did not have a significantly different length of survival than those expressing a normal constellation of antigens.

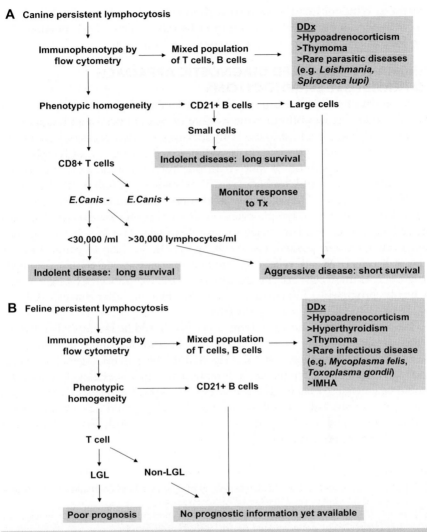

Fig. 1. (A) Algorithm for the workup of cases of canine persistent lymphocytosis. (B) Algorithm for the workup of cases of feline persistent lymphocytosis. DDX, differential diagnosis; IMHA, immune mediated hemolytic anemia; Tx, therapy.

Prognosis in Feline Neoplastic Lymphocytosis

There are no studies correlating the immunophenotype with outcome in feline neoplastic lymphocytosis, although two recent reports may help with prognostication in some cases. Workman and colleagues [57] found a wide range of survival in cats with CD4+ CLL, with a mean of 28 months in treated cases. By contrast, LGL malignancy in cats, which is most commonly CD8+, can present as lymphocytosis associated with intestinal lymphoma [86,87]. These cases have a poor survival time (mean of 84 days). Thus, LGL phenotype is one feature that seems to provide prognostic information.

SUMMARY: PROPOSED DIAGNOSTIC APPROACH TO PERSISTENT LYMPHOCYTOSIS

Based on data from the literature and the authors' clinical experience, they propose the following algorithm for the workup of cases of persistent lymphocytosis (Fig. 1A). Dogs with absolute lymphocytosis on two occasions should be immunophenotyped. Those animals with a mixed population of lymphocytes (defined by an expansion of more than one subset) should be evaluated for nonneoplastic causes of lymphocytosis. These patients should be in the minority. Most dogs have a homogeneous population (in the authors' experience, the expanded population of lymphocytes consistently comprises greater than 80% of the lymphocytes) and are likely to have neoplasia. The presence of an aberrant phenotype or a positive test result by PARR can help to confirm this. If these cells are CD8+ T cells, the lymphocyte count at presentation is highly prognostic. If these cells are B cells, the size of the lymphocytes by light scatter is highly prognostic. Information about survival in other subsets (CD4+, CD4−CD8−CD5+) is not yet available.

Cats with repeatable absolute lymphocytosis should be immunophenotyped. If their lymphocytes are heterogeneous, they should be evaluated for nonneoplastic causes of lymphocytosis (see Fig. 1B). If there is homogeneous expansion of lymphocytes, leukemia or lymphoma with circulating lymphocytes should be considered likely. The immunophenotype of neoplastic lymphocytes is not yet prognostically useful in cats, but the cells should be carefully examined to determine if the lymphocytes have an LGL morphology. These cases seem to have a poor outcome.

References

[1] Barr SC, Van Beek O, Carlisle-Nowak MS, et al. *Trypanosoma cruzi* infection in Walker hounds from Virginia. Am J Vet Res 1995;56:1037–44.

[2] Meurs KM, Anthony MA, Slater M, et al. Chronic *Trypanosoma cruzi* infection in dogs: 11 cases (1987-1996). J Am Vet Med Assoc 1998;213:497–500.

[3] Inokuma H, Okuda M, Yoshizaki Y, et al. Clinical observations of *Babesia gibsoni* infection with low parasitaemia confirmed by PCR in dogs. Vet Rec 2005;156:116–8.

[4] Meinkoth JH, Kocan AA, Loud SD, et al. Clinical and hematologic effects of experimental infection of dogs with recently identified *Babesia gibsoni*-like isolates from Oklahoma. J Am Vet Med Assoc 2002;220:185–9.

[5] Bastos Cde V, Moreira SM, Passos LM. Retrospective study (1998-2001) on canine babesiosis in Belo Horizonte, Minas Gerais, Brazil. Ann N Y Acad Sci 2004;1026:158–60.

[6] Panciera RJ, Ewing SA, Mathew JS, et al. Canine hepatozoonosis: comparison of lesions and parasites in skeletal muscle of dogs experimentally or naturally infected with *Hepatozoon americanum*. Vet Parasitol 1999;82:261–72.

[7] Rosypal AC, Troy GC, Duncan RB, et al. Utility of diagnostic tests used in diagnosis of infection in dogs experimentally inoculated with a North American isolate of *Leishmania infantum infantum*. J Vet Intern Med 2005;19:802–9.

[8] Gaskin AA, Schantz P, Jackson J, et al. Visceral leishmaniasis in a New York foxhound kennel. J Vet Intern Med 2002;16:34–44.

[9] Mylonakis ME, Rallis T, Koutinas AF, et al. Clinical signs and clinicopathologic abnormalities in dogs with clinical spirocercosis: 39 cases (1996-2004). J Am Vet Med Assoc 2006; 228:1063–7.

[10] Sharma MC, Pachauri SP. Blood cellular and biochemical studies in canine dirofilariasis. Vet Res Commun 1982;5:295–300.

[11] Mikszewski JS, Vite CH. Central nervous system dysfunction associated with Rocky Mountain Spotted Fever infection in five dogs. J Am Anim Hosp Assoc 2005;41:259–66.

[12] Breitschwerdt EB, Davidson MG, Hegarty BC, et al. Prednisolone at anti-inflammatory or immunosuppressive dosages in conjunction with doxycycline does not potentiate the severity of Rickettsia rickettsii infection in dogs. Antimicrob Agents Chemother 1997;41:141–7.

[13] Egenvall AE, Hedhammar AA, Bjoersdorff AI. Clinical features and serology of 14 dogs affected by granulocytic ehrlichiosis in Sweden. Vet Rec 1997;140:222–6.

[14] Lilliehook I, Egenvall A, Tvedten HW. Hematopathology in dogs experimentally infected with a Swedish granulocytic Ehrlichia species. Vet Clin Pathol 1998;27:116–22.

[15] Codner EC, Farris-Smith LL. Characterization of the subclinical phase of ehrlichiosis in dogs. J Am Vet Med Assoc 1986;189:47–50.

[16] Heeb HL, Wilkerson MJ, Chun R, et al. Large granular lymphocytosis, lymphocyte subset inversion, thrombocytopenia, dysproteinemia, and positive Ehrlichia serology in a dog. J Am Anim Hosp Assoc 2003;39:379–84.

[17] Weiser MG, Thrall MA, Fulton R, et al. Granular lymphocytosis and hyperproteinemia in dogs with chronic ehrlichiosis. J Am Anim Hosp Assoc 1991;27:84–8.

[18] Frank JR, Breitschwerdt EB. A retrospective study of ehrlichiosis in 62 dogs from North Carolina and Virginia. J Vet Intern Med 1999;13:194–201.

[19] Kuehn NF, Gaunt SD. Clinical and hematologic findings in canine ehrlichiosis. J Am Vet Med Assoc 1985;186:355–8.

[20] Breitschwerdt EB, Hegarty BC, Hancock SI. Sequential evaluation of dogs naturally infected with Ehrlichia canis, Ehrlichia chaffeensis, Ehrlichia equi, Ehrlichia ewingii, or Bartonella vinsonii. J Clin Microbiol 1998;36:2645–51.

[21] McDonough SP, Moore PF. Clinical, hematologic, and immunophenotypic characterization of canine large granular lymphocytosis. Vet Pathol 2000;37:637–46.

[22] Hess PR, English RV, Hegarty BC, et al. Experimental Ehrlichia canis infection in the dog does not cause immunosuppression. Vet Immunol Immunopathol 2005;117–25.

[23] Birkenheuer AJ, Le JA, Valenzisi AM, et al. Cytauxzoon felis infection in cats in the mid-Atlantic states: 34 cases (1998-2004). J Am Vet Med Assoc 2006;228:568–71.

[24] Peterson JL, Willard MD, Lees GE, et al. Toxoplasmosis in two cats with inflammatory intestinal disease. J Am Vet Med Assoc 1991;199:473–6.

[25] Lappin MR, Breitschwerdt EB, Jensen WA, et al. Molecular and serologic evidence of Anaplasma phagocytophilum infection in cats in North America. J Am Vet Med Assoc 2004;225:893–6.

[26] Atkins CE, DeFrancesco TC, Coats JR, et al. Heartworm infection in cats: 50 cases (1985-1997). J Am Vet Med Assoc 2000;217:355–8.

[27] Westfall DS, Jensen WA, Reagan WJ, et al. Inoculation of two genotypes of Hemobartonella felis (California and Ohio variants) to induce infection in cats and the response to treatment with azithromycin. Am J Vet Res 2001;62:687–91.

[28] Lappin MR, George JW, Pedersen NC, et al. Primary and secondary Toxoplasma gondii infection in normal and feline immunodeficiency virus-infected cats. J Parasitol 1996;82:733–42.

[29] Harrus S, Klement E, Aroch I, et al. Retrospective study of 46 cases of feline haemobartonellosis in Israel and their relationships with FeLV and FIV infections. Vet Rec 2002;151:82–5.

[30] Breitschwerdt EB, Abrams-Ogg AC, Lappin MR, et al. Molecular evidence supporting Ehrlichia canis-like infection in cats. J Vet Intern Med 2002;16:642–9.

[31] Shelton GH, Linenberger ML. Hematologic abnormalities associated with retroviral infections in the cat. Semin Vet Med Surg (Small Anim) 1995;10:220–33.

[32] Hopper CD, Sparkes AH, Gruffydd-Jones TJ, et al. Clinical and laboratory findings in cats infected with feline immunodeficiency virus. Vet Rec 1989;125:341–6.

[33] Weinkle TK, Center SA, Randolph JF, et al. Evaluation of prognostic factors, survival rates, and treatment protocols for immune-mediated hemolytic anemia in dogs: 151 cases (1993-2002). J Am Vet Med Assoc 2005;226:1869–80.

[34] Thompson MF, Scott-Moncrieff JC, Brooks MB. Effect of a single plasma transfusion on thromboembolism in 13 dogs with primary immune-mediated hemolytic anemia. J Am Anim Hosp Assoc 2004;40:446–54.

[35] Mason N, Duval D, Shofer FS, et al. Cyclophosphamide exerts no beneficial effect over prednisone alone in the initial treatment of acute immune-mediated hemolytic anemia in dogs: a randomized controlled clinical trial. J Vet Intern Med 2003;17:206–12.

[36] Kohn B, Weingart C, Eckmann V, et al. Primary immune-mediated hemolytic anemia in 19 cats: diagnosis, therapy, and outcome (1998-2004). J Vet Intern Med 2006;20:159–66.

[37] Weiss DJ. Differentiating benign and malignant causes of lymphocytosis in feline bone marrow. J Vet Intern Med 2005;19:855–9.

[38] Chabanne L, Fournel C, Caux C, et al. Abnormalities of lymphocyte subsets in canine systemic lupus erythematosus. Autoimmunity 1995;22:1–8.

[39] Rondeau MP, Walton RM, Bissett S, et al. Suppurative, nonseptic polyarthropathy in dogs. J Vet Intern Med 2005;19:654–62.

[40] Melian C, Peterson ME. Diagnosis and treatment of naturally occurring hypoadrenocorticism in 42 dogs. J Small Anim Pract 1996;37:268–75.

[41] Peterson ME, Kintzer PP, Kass PH. Pretreatment clinical and laboratory findings in dogs with hypoadrenocorticism: 225 cases (1979-1993). J Am Vet Med Assoc 1996;208: 85–91.

[42] Rakich PM, Lorenz MD. Clinical signs and laboratory abnormalities in 23 dogs with spontaneous hypoadrenocorticism. J Am Anim Hosp Assoc 1984;20:647–9.

[43] Lifton SJ, King LG, Zerbe CA. Glucocorticoid deficient hypoadrenocorticism in dogs: 18 cases (1986-1995). J Am Vet Med Assoc 1996;209:2076–81.

[44] Peterson ME, Greco DS, Orth DN. Primary hypoadrenocorticism in ten cats. J Vet Intern Med 1989;3:55–8.

[45] Thoday KL, Mooney CT. Historical, clinical and laboratory features of 126 hyperthyroid cats. Vet Rec 1992;131:257–64.

[46] Peterson ME, Kintzer PP, Hurvitz AI. Methimazole treatment of 262 cats with hyperthyroidism. J Vet Intern Med 1988;2:150–7.

[47] Barton AD. T-cell lymphocytosis associated with lymphocyte-rich thymoma. Cancer 1997; 80:1409–17.

[48] Atwater SW, Powers BE, Park RD, et al. Thymoma in dogs: 23 cases (1980-1991). J Am Vet Med Assoc 1994;205:1007–13.

[49] Bellah JR, Stiff ME, Russell RG. Thymoma in the dog: two case reports and review of 20 additional cases. J Am Vet Med Assoc 1983;183:306–11.

[50] Lana S, Plaza S, Hampe R, et al. Diagnosis of mediastinal masses in dogs by flow cytometry. J Vet Intern Med 2006;20:1161–5.

[51] Phillips TR, Jensen JL, Rubino MJ, et al. Effects of vaccines on the canine immune system. Can J Vet Res 1989;53:154–60.

[52] Miyamoto T, Taura Y, Une S, et al. Immunological responses to polyvalent canine vaccines in dogs. J Vet Med Sci 1995;57:347–9.

[53] McMillen GL, Briggs DJ, McVey DS, et al. Vaccination of racing greyhounds: effects on humoral and cellular immunity. Vet Immunol Immunopathol 1995;49:101–13.

[54] Vernau W, Moore PF. An immunophenotypic study of canine leukemias and preliminary assessment of clonality by polymerase chain reaction. Vet Immunol Immunopathol 1999;69: 145–64.

[55] Leifer CE, Matus RE. Chronic lymphocytic leukemia in the dog: 22 cases (1974-1984). J Am Vet Med Assoc 1986;189:214–7.

[56] Workman HC, Vernau W. Chronic lymphocytic leukemia in dogs and cats: the veterinary perspective. Vet Clin North Am Small Anim Pract 2003;33:1379–99.

[57] Workman HC, Vernau W, Schmidt PS, et al. Chronic lymphocytic leukemia in cats is primarily a T helper cell disease. Presented at the 55th Annual Meeting of the American College of Veterinary Pathologists. Orlando, November 13–17, 2004.

[58] Keller RL, Avery AC, Burnett RC, et al. Detection of neoplastic lymphocytes in peripheral blood of dogs with lymphoma by polymerase chain reaction for antigen receptor gene rearrangement. Vet Clin Pathol 2004;33:145–9.

[59] Raskin RE, Krehbiel JD. Prevalence of leukemic blood and bone marrow in dogs with multicentric lymphoma. J Am Vet Med Assoc 1989;194:1427–9.

[60] Appelbaum FR, Sale GE, Storb R, et al. Phenotyping of canine lymphoma with monoclonal antibodies directed at cell surface antigens: classification, morphology, clinical presentation and response to chemotherapy. Hematol Oncol 1984;2:151–68.

[61] Madewell BR. Hematologic and bone marrow cytologic abnormalities in 75 dogs with malignant lymphoma. J Am Anim Hosp Assoc 1986;22:235–40.

[62] Gabor LJ, Canfield PJ, Malik R. Haematological and biochemical findings in cats in Australia with lymphosarcoma. Aust Vet J 2000;78:456–61.

[63] Davis BH, Foucar K, Szczarkowski W, et al. U.S.-Canadian consensus recommendations on the immunophenotypic analysis of hematologic neoplasia by flow cytometry: medical indications. Cytometry 1997;30:249–63.

[64] Avery PR, Avery AC. Molecular methods to distinguish reactive and neoplastic lymphocyte expansions and their importance in transitional neoplastic states. Vet Clin Pathol 2004;33: 196–207.

[65] Lindblad-Toh K, Lander ES, Mikkelsen TS, et al. Genome sequence, comparative analysis and haplotype structure of the domestic dog. Nature 2005;438:803–19.

[66] Kirkness EF, Bafna V, Halpern AL, et al. The dog genome: survey sequencing and comparative analysis. Science 2003;301:1898–903.

[67] Thomas R, Smith KC, Ostrander EA, et al. Chromosome aberrations in canine multicentric lymphomas detected with comparative genomic hybridisation and a panel of single locus probes. Br J Cancer 2003;89:1530–7.

[68] Dean GA. Antigens and immunophenotyping. 5th edition. Lippincott, Baltimore (MD): Schalm's Veterinary Hematology; 2000.

[69] Ruslander DA, Gebhard DH, Tompkins MB, et al. Immunophenotypic characterization of canine lymphoproliferative disorders. In vivo 1997;11:169–72.

[70] Modiano JF, Breen M, Burnett RC, et al. Distinct B-cell and T-cell lymphoproliferative disease prevalence among dog breeds indicates heritable risk. Cancer Res 2005;65: 5654–61.

[71] Schabath R, Ratei R, Ludwig WD. The prognostic significance of antigen expression in leukaemia. Baillieres Best Pract Res Clin Haematol 2003;16:613–28.

[72] Rezuke WN, Abernathy EC, Tsongalis GJ. Molecular diagnosis of B- and T-cell lymphomas: fundamental principles and clinical applications. Clin Chem 1997;43: 1814–23.

[73] Jennings CD, Foon KA. Recent advances in flow cytometry: application to the diagnosis of hematologic malignancy. Blood 1997;90:2863–92.

[74] Gorczyca W, Tugulea S, Liu Z, et al. Flow cytometry in the diagnosis of mediastinal tumors with emphasis on differentiating thymocytes from precursor T-lymphoblastic lymphoma/leukemia. Leuk Lymphoma 2004;45:529–38.

[75] Kamihira S, Sohda H, Atogami S, et al. Phenotypic diversity and prognosis of adult T-cell leukemia. Leuk Res 1992;16:435–41.

[76] Uckun FM, Gaynon PS, Sensel MG, et al. Clinical features and treatment outcome of childhood T-lineage acute lymphoblastic leukemia according to the apparent maturational stage

of T-lineage leukemic blasts: a Children's Cancer Group study. J Clin Oncol 1997;15: 2214–21.

[77] Czuczman MS, Dodge RK, Stewart CC, et al. Value of immunophenotype in intensively treated adult acute lymphoblastic leukemia: cancer and leukemia Group B study 8364. Blood 1999;93:3931–9.

[78] Avery PR, Williams M, Avery AC. Canine lymphocytic leukemia: are there prognostic markers? Presented at the American College of Veterinary Internal Medicine Forum. Louisville, May 31–June 3, 2006.

[79] Burnett RC, Vernau W, Modiano JF, et al. Diagnosis of canine lymphoid neoplasia using clonal rearrangements of antigen receptor genes. Vet Pathol 2003;40:32–41.

[80] Swerdlow SH. Genetic and molecular genetic studies in the diagnosis of atypical lymphoid hyperplasias versus lymphoma. Hum Pathol 2003;34:346–51.

[81] Matutes E, Owusu-Ankomah K, Morilla R, et al. The immunological profile of B-cell disorders and proposal of a scoring system for the diagnosis of CLL. Leukemia 1994;8:1640–5.

[82] Greenlee PG, Filippa DA, Quimby FW, et al. Lymphomas in dogs. Cancer 1990;66: 480–90.

[83] Teske E. Canine malignant lymphoma: a review and comparison with human non-Hodgkin's lymphoma. Vet Q 1994;4:209–19.

[84] Herishanu Y, Polliack A. Chronic lymphocytic leukemia: a review of some new aspects of the biology, factors influencing prognosis and therapeutic options. Transfus Apher Sci 2005; 32:85–97.

[85] Nenova I, Mateva N, Ananoshtev N, et al. The prognostic value of clinical and laboratory parameters in patients with chronic lymphocytic leukemia. Hematology 2005;10:47–51.

[86] Roccabianca P, Vernau W, Caniatti M, et al. Feline large granular lymphocyte (LGL) lymphoma with secondary leukemia: primary intestinal origin with predominance of a CD3/CD8αα phenotype. Vet Pathol 2006;43:15–28.

[87] Wellman ML, Hammer AS, DiBartola SP, et al. Lymphoma involving large granular lymphocytes in cats: 11 cases (1982-1991). J Am Vet Med Assoc 1992;201:1265–9.

Vet Clin Small Anim 37 (2007) 283–295

VETERINARY CLINICS
SMALL ANIMAL PRACTICE

Measurement, Interpretation, and Implications of Proteinuria and Albuminuria

Gregory F. Grauer, DVM, MS

Department of Clinical Sciences, College of Veterinary Medicine, 111B Mosier Hall, Kansas State University, Manhattan, KS 66506, USA

Persistent proteinuria of renal origin is an important marker of chronic kidney disease (CKD) in dogs and cats. Unfortunately, because of the high incidence of false-positive results for proteinuria on the urine dipstick screening test and proteinuria associated with lower urinary tract inflammation in dogs and cats, positive reactions for urine protein are quite common, and therefore often disregarded. Ruling out false-positive proteinuria and identifying proteinuria of renal origin are necessary first steps when evaluating the results of tests for proteinuria. In the case of CKD, albumin is usually the primary component of renal proteinuria. In addition to being a diagnostic marker for CKD, the potential for renal proteinuria/albuminuria to be a mediator of CKD progression also exists. The recent development of species-specific albumin ELISA technology that enables detection of low concentrations of canine and feline albuminuria has stimulated discussion about what level of proteinuria/albuminuria is normal and what levels may be associated with renal disease progression. For these reasons, detection and monitoring of renal proteinuria in dogs and cats have recently received renewed interest. Perhaps somewhat similar to our changing definition and treatment guidelines for systemic hypertension, the need to recognize, monitor, and potentially treat renal proteinuria, which may have been considered normal not long ago, is increasing.

NORMAL PHYSIOLOGY

The urine of healthy dogs and cats contains only a small amount of albumin and other proteins. The selective permeability of the glomerular capillary wall restricts the filtration of most plasma proteins, primarily on the basis of protein weight and, to a lesser extent, on the basis of protein charge size, and sterical configuration. Small and electrically neutral or positively charged proteins are more readily filtered than are large and negatively charged

E-mail address: ggrauer@vet.k-state.edu

0195-5616/07/$ – see front matter
doi:10.1016/j.cvsm.2006.11.003

proteins. For example, normal glomerular filtrate usually contains little protein with a molecular weight the size of albumin (69,000 d) or greater.

The glomerular capillary wall has three primary components: the endothelial cells that line the capillary lumen, the basement membrane, and the epithelial cells that line the visceral surface of the capillary wall (Fig. 1). The endothelial cells are highly fenestrated and provide part of the electrostatic barrier for negatively charged proteins. The basement membrane is composed of hydrated and tightly cross-linked type IV collagen, laminin, nidogen, and proteoglycans. Glomerular epithelial cells, also known as podocytes, form extensions (foot processes) that interdigitate on the visceral surface of the basement membrane. These podocyte foot processes are covered by a proteinaceous structure known as the slit diaphragm. The glomerular basement membrane and the slit diaphragm are thought provide most of the size- and charge-selective permeability of the glomerular capillary wall.

The glomerular filtrate of healthy dogs and cats contains only 2 to 3 mg/dL of albumin compared with the 4 g/dL of albumin found in the plasma. Smaller molecular-weight proteins as well as those positively charged larger proteins that do pass through the glomerular capillary wall are almost completely reabsorbed by tubular epithelial cells by an active process termed *pinocytosis*. Such reabsorbed proteins may be broken down and used by the epithelial cells or returned to the bloodstream. This protein reabsorption occurs primarily in the proximal convoluted tubule and reduces the concentration of albumin in normal distal tubular fluid to less than 1 mg/dL. This reabsorptive process has a transport maximum, however. Tubular proteinuria may occur if that maximum is exceeded (eg, excessive production of small-molecular-weight proteins like Bence-Jones proteins) or if damage to the tubular epithelial cells

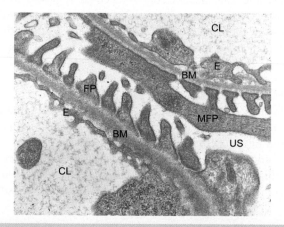

Fig. 1. Transmission electron micrograph of the glomerular capillary wall from a normal dog. BM, basement membrane; CL, capillary lumen; E, endothelial cell (note fenestrations); FP, podocyte foot processes; MFP, major foot process; US, urinary space.

(eg, nephrotoxic damage, chronic tubulointerstitial disease) decreases their reabsorptive capacity.

Protein present in normal urine may also result from the secretion of enzymes, mucoproteins, and immunoglobulins by tubular and lower urinary and genital tract epithelial cells. These secreted proteins may account for as much as 50% of the proteins that are present in the urine of healthy animals.

SCREENING TESTS FOR PROTEINURIA

Proteinuria is routinely detected by semiquantitative screening methods, such as the conventional dipstick colorimetric test (common) and the sulfosalicylic acid (SSA) turbidimetric test (less common). The dipstick test is inexpensive and easy to use (Fig. 2). This test primarily measures albumin; however, the sensitivity and specificity for albumin are relatively low with the dipstick methodology. False-negative results (decreased sensitivity) may occur in the setting of Bence-Jones proteinuria, low concentrations of urine albumin, or dilute or acidic urine. The conventional dipstick test has a sensitivity level of greater than 30 mg/dL. False-positive results (decreased specificity) may be obtained if the urine is alkaline or highly concentrated, the urine sediment is active (pyuria, hematuria, or bacteriuria), or the dipstick is left in contact with the urine long enough to leach out the citrate buffer that is incorporated in the filter paper pad. False-positive results with the dipstick method occur more frequently in cats compared with dogs but are common in both species. For example, when 298 canine and feline urine samples were analyzed by a conventional urine protein dipstick method (Multistix Reagent Strips; Bayer Corporation, Elkhart, Indiana) and a canine or feline albumin-specific quantitative ELISA (Heska Corporation, Fort Collins, Colorado), there were disparate results [1]. The sensitivity for the conventional urine protein dipstick test for albuminuria in canine and feline urine was 54% and 60%, respectively, and the urine

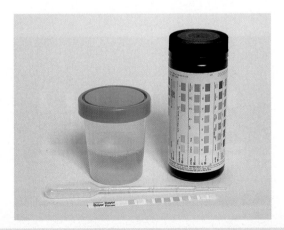

Fig. 2. Standard screening with dipstick methodology for assessment of proteinuria.

protein dipstick specificity for canine and feline albuminuria was 69% and 31%, respectively. If urine samples with an alkaline pH ($\geq$7.5) or hematuria ($\geq$10 red blood cells [RBCs] per high-power field [hpf]), pyuria ($\geq$5 white blood cells [WBCs]/hpf), or bacteriuria were excluded, the dipstick specificity for canine and feline albuminuria increased to 84% and 55%, respectively. These data demonstrate that conventional urine protein dipstick tests have a high percentage of false-negative and false-positive results for detection of albuminuria in canine and feline urine when compared with an albumin-specific ELISA. Urine protein dipstick false-positive results in both species can be decreased by excluding alkaline urine and urine with hematuria, pyuria, or bacteriuria from analysis.

The SSA test is performed by mixing equal quantities of urine supernatant and 5% SSA in a glass test tube and grading the turbidity that results from precipitation of protein on a scale from 0 to 4+ (Fig. 3). In addition to albumin, the SSA test can detect globulins and Bence-Jones proteins. False-positive results may occur if the urine contains radiographic contrast agents, penicillin, cephalosporins, sulfisoxazole, or the urine preservative thymol. The protein content may also be overestimated with the SSA test if uncentrifuged turbid urine is analyzed. False-negative results are less common in comparison with the conventional dipstick test because of the increased sensitivity of the SSA test for protein (>5 mg/dL). Because of the relatively poor specificity of the conventional dipstick analysis, many reference laboratories confirm a positive dipstick test result for proteinuria with the SSA test. Grading of the color change on the dipstick test and the turbidity on the SSA test is subjective; therefore, results can vary between individuals and laboratories.

Proteinuria detected by these semiquantitative screening methods has historically been interpreted in light of the urine specific gravity and urine sediment. For example, a positive dipstick reading of trace or 1+ proteinuria in hypersthenuric urine has often been attributed to urine concentration rather than

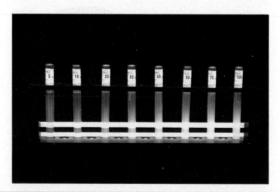

Fig. 3. SSA standards demonstrate the increasing turbidity that occurs with increasing proteinuria when 5% SSA is mixed with an equal volume of urine.

to abnormal proteinuria. In addition, a positive dipstick reading for protein in the presence of microscopic hematuria or pyuria has often been attributed to urinary tract hemorrhage or inflammation. In both examples, the interpretation may not be correct. Given the limits of the conventional dipstick test sensitivity, any positive result for protein, regardless of urine concentration, may be abnormal (except in the case of false-positive results). Likewise, hematuria and pyuria have an inconsistent effect on urine albumin concentrations; not all dogs with hematuria and pyuria have albuminuria [2].

LOCALIZATION OF PROTEINURIA

When proteinuria is detected by screening tests, it is important to try to identify its source. Proteinuria may be caused by physiologic or pathologic conditions (Table 1). Physiologic or benign proteinuria is often transient and abates when the underlying cause is corrected. Strenuous exercise, seizures, fever, exposure to extreme heat or cold, and stress are examples of conditions that may cause physiologic proteinuria. The mechanism of physiologic proteinuria is not completely understood; however, transient renal vasoconstriction, ischemia, and congestion are thought to be involved. Decreased physical activity may also affect urine protein excretion in dogs; one study showed that urinary protein loss was higher in dogs confined to cages than in dogs with normal activity levels [3].

Pathologic proteinuria may be caused by urinary or nonurinary abnormalities. Nonurinary disorders associated with proteinuria often involve the production of small-molecular-weight proteins (dysproteinemias) that are filtered by the glomeruli and subsequently overwhelm the reabsorptive capacity of the proximal tubule. An example of this "prerenal" proteinuria is the production of immunoglobulin light chains (Bence-Jones proteins) by neoplastic plasma cells. Genital tract inflammation (eg, prostatitis, metritis) can also result in pathologic nonurinary proteinuria. Obtaining urine samples by means of cystocentesis reduces the potential for urine contamination with protein from the lower urinary tract.

Pathologic urinary proteinuria may be renal or nonrenal in origin. Nonrenal proteinuria most frequently occurs in association with lower urinary tract inflammation or hemorrhage (also referred to as postrenal proteinuria). Changes observed in the urine sediment are usually compatible with the underlying inflammation (eg, pyuria, hematuria, bacteriuria, increased numbers of transitional epithelial cells). Conversely, renal proteinuria is most often caused by increased glomerular filtration of plasma proteins associated with intraglomerular hypertension or the presence of immune complexes, structural damage, or vascular inflammation in the glomerular capillaries. Renal proteinuria may also be caused by decreased reabsorption of filtered plasma proteins attributable to tubulointerstitial disease. In some cases, tubulointerstitial proteinuria may be accompanied by normoglycemic glucosuria and increased excretion of electrolytes (eg, Fanconi syndrome, acute tubular damage). Glomerular lesions usually result in higher magnitude proteinuria compared with proteinuria

Table 1
Localization of proteinuria

Type of proteinuria		Diagnosis
Physiologic/benign proteinuria		UP/C usually <0.5 Compatible history Intermittent/transient
Examples include	Change in exercise level Seizure activity Fever Exposure to temperature extremes Stress	
Pathologic proteinuria Nonurinary		Variable UP/C
Examples include	Congestive heart failure	History/PE/ echocardiogram
	Hemoglobinuria/ myoglobinuria	Urine remains red after centrifugation
	Dysproteinemia/ dysproteinuria	Serum/urine electrophoresis
	Genital tract inflammation/ hemorrhage	PE/imaging/urine sediment
Urinary, nonrenal Examples include	Lower urinary tract inflammation (eg, bacterial cystitis, cystoliths, polyps, neoplasia)	UP/C not indicated History/PE Urine sediment Imaging
Urinary, renal Examples include	Renal parenchymal inflammation (eg, pyelonephritis, renoliths, neoplasia)	Variable UP/C Urine sediment Imaging
	Tubular proteinuria	UP/C usually 0.5–1.0 Can be associated with normoglycemic glucosuria and excessive urinary loss of electrolytes
	Glomerular proteinuria	Persistent UP/C $\geq$1.0 Inactive urine sediment with the exception of possible hyaline casts

Abbreviations: PE, physical exam; UP/C, urine protein/creatinine ratio.

associated with tubulointerstitial lesions. Renal proteinuria caused by glomerular and tubular disease is most frequently accompanied by an inactive urine sediment, with the exception being the presence of hyaline casts. In addition to glomerular and tubulointerstitial disease, renal proteinuria may be caused by inflammatory or infiltrative disorders of the kidney (eg, neoplasia, pyelonephritis, leptospirosis), which are often accompanied by an active urine sediment.

DETECTION OF ALBUMINURIA/MICROALBUMINURIA

Albuminuria can be measured by point-of-care semiquantitative tests (eg, E.R.D.-HealthScreen Urine test; Heska Corporation) and quantitative immunoassays at reference laboratories. Like proteinuria, albuminuria can be caused by pre- and postrenal disorders; therefore, it is important to localize the source of albuminuria as discussed previously. Microalbuminuria (MA) is defined as concentrations of albumin in the urine that are greater than normal but less than the limit of detection using conventional dipstick urine protein screening methodology (ie, ≤30 mg/dL). Urine albumin concentrations greater than 30 mg/dL are referred to as overt albuminuria and can often be detected using the urine protein/creatinine ratio (UP/C) (see section on quantitation of proteinuria). The lower end of the MA range has been less easily defined because of the requirement that this concentration be greater than "normal" and the necessity that this concentration be reliably detected. In the dog and cat, the lower limit was defined based on the log mean plus 2 standard deviations of populations of apparently healthy dogs and cats as greater than 1 mg/dL. Urine albumin concentrations can be adjusted for differences in urine concentration by dividing by urine creatinine concentrations. For example, a urine albumin/creatinine ratio greater than 0.03 is considered abnormal in people. Alternatively, urine can be diluted to a standard concentration, such as 1.010, before assay. In one study of dogs, normalizing urine albumin concentrations to a 1.010 specific gravity yielded similar results to the urine albumin/creatinine ratio [4].

Indications for the use of MA tests [5] include the following: (1) when conventional screening tests for proteinuria produce equivocal or conflicting results or false-positive results are suspected, (2) when conventional screening tests for proteinuria are negative in apparently healthy older dogs and cats and a more sensitive screening test is desired, (3) when conventional screening tests for proteinuria are negative in apparently healthy young dogs and cats with a familial risk for developing proteinuric renal disease and a more sensitive screening test is desired, (4) when conventional screening test results for proteinuria are negative in dogs and cats with chronic illnesses that are associated with proteinuria renal disease and a more sensitive screening test is desired, 5) when a previous MA test result(s) was positive and monitoring for persistence or progression of the MA is desired.

CAUSES OF MICROALBUMINURIA

MA reflects the presence of intraglomerular hypertension or generalized vascular damage and endothelial cell dysfunction in human beings [6]. It is interesting to note that the presence of MA has been shown to be an accurate predictor of subsequent renal disease in human beings with systemic hypertension and diabetes mellitus, and it has also been observed in human beings with systemic diseases that are associated with glomerulopathy [7–11]. Importantly, early detection of albuminuria and institution of appropriate treatment have slowed the progression of kidney disease in people [12].

Based on recent studies, MA seems to be a good indicator of early renal disease in dogs, particularly those diseases that involve the glomerulus [4,13,14]. Albuminuria was evaluated in 36 male dogs with X-linked hereditary nephropathy, a rapidly progressive glomerular disease that is secondary to a defect in type IV collagen, a structural component of the glomerular basement membrane [4]. In these dogs, lesions in the glomerular basement membrane become apparent by 8 weeks of age. Persistent MA was detected between 8 and 23 weeks of age, 0 to 16 weeks before the onset of overt proteinuria, which occurred at 14 to 30 weeks of age. It was concluded that MA was a reliable early marker of developing nephropathy.

In 12 healthy dogs that were experimentally infected with *Dirofilaria immitis* L3 larvae and longitudinally evaluated, all the dogs developed MA, with 82% of all samples collected over the 14- to 23-month postinfection period of study being positive for MA [13]. The onset of MA corresponded to the onset of antigenemia. The magnitude of MA increased over time, and MA preceded the development of overt proteinuria, as measured by the UP/C. At the end of the study, the dogs had histologic evidence of glomerular disease by light (n = 11) or electron (n = 12) microscopy [13].

Finally, the prevalence of MA in 20 Soft-Coated Wheaten Terriers that were genetically at risk for the development of protein-losing enteropathy and nephropathy was 76% [14]. The magnitude of MA increased over time, and 43% of the dogs with MA eventually developed abnormal UP/Cs. Of interest is the observation that persistent MA develops in dogs with this type of protein-losing nephropathy at approximately the same time that mesangial hypercellularity and segmental glomerular sclerosis occur. Concurrent inflammatory bowel disease may account for MA in some of the dogs that have not progressed to overt proteinuria.

Other conditions have been reported in dogs with MA, including infectious, inflammatory, neoplastic, metabolic, and cardiovascular disease [15,16]. Results of a study of MA in dogs with lymphosarcoma and osteosarcoma demonstrated that urine albumin concentrations were significantly increased in dogs with these tumors, even though the UP/Cs may not be increased to greater than the reference range [17]. Urine albumin concentrations did not, however, consistently decrease with decreased tumor burden.

The prevalence of MA in dogs admitted to intensive care unit (ICU) is higher than in other reported patient populations and seems to vary with different classifications of disease [15,16]. As reported in people with acute inflammatory conditions, transient MA occurred in some of these dogs. A large percentage of patients that were euthanized or died had MA, suggesting that, as in people, the presence of MA may be a negative prognostic indicator.

Although amoxicillin and clavulanic acid and carprofen do not seem to affect albuminuria, corticosteroid administration does increase albuminuria. Short-term prednisone administration has been shown to cause a substantial but reversible increase in the magnitude of proteinuria in heterozygous, or carrier, female dogs with X-linked hereditary nephropathy [18]. Finally, a moderate amount of exercise (treadmill work for 20 minutes) did not affect albuminuria in dogs [19].

It is important to note that the sensitivity of MA assays makes it likely that some positive results are caused by benign or physiologic proteinuria. In these cases, follow-up assays should be negative, confirming that the MA was transient. Transient MA is likely to be of little or no consequence.

QUANTITATION OF PROTEINURIA

If the results of the screening tests suggest the presence of renal proteinuria/albuminuria, urine protein excretion should be quantified. This helps to evaluate the severity of renal lesions and to assess the response to treatment or the progression of disease. Methods used to quantitate proteinuria include the UP/C and immunoassays for albuminuria, the results of which are expressed as urine albumin/creatinine ratios or in milligrams per deciliter in urine samples that have been diluted to a standard urine specific gravity (eg, 1.010). Albumin greater than or equal to 30 mg/dL in urine that has been diluted to a specific gravity of 1.010 usually results in UP/Cs greater than the normal range in cats and dogs. Urine that contains enough albumin to register greater than a medium reaction on the early renal damage (ERD) test also often has a UP/C greater than the normal range. The UP/C and urine albumin/creatinine ratio from spot urine samples have been shown to reflect the quantity of protein/albumin excreted in the urine over a 24-hour period accurately. Because of the difficulty of 24-hour urine collection, this methodology has greatly facilitated the diagnosis of proteinuric renal disease in veterinary medicine. Most studies have shown that normal urine protein excretion in dogs and cats is 10 to 30 mg/kg or less over 24 hours and that normal UP/Cs are 0.2 to 0.3 or less [20–22]. Initially recommended normal values for canine UP/Cs of less than 1.0 were likely conservative and have more recently been lowered. Today, UP/Cs less than 0.5 and less than 0.4 are considered to be normal for dogs and cats, respectively [5]. Persistent proteinuria that results in UP/Cs greater than 0.4 and greater than 0.5 in cats and dogs, respectively, in which pre- and postrenal proteinuria has been ruled out, are consistent with glomerular or tubulointerstitial CKD. UP/Cs greater than 2.0 are strongly suggestive of glomerular disease. The definition of normal may continue to change with additional research. For example, even the ultralow-level single-nephron proteinuria that can arise secondary to intraglomerular hypertension in hypertrophied nephrons in CKD is abnormal in the face of what may be considered normal whole-body or whole-kidney proteinuria.

MONITORING RENAL PROTEINURIA

Transient renal proteinuria/albuminuria is likely of little consequence and does not warrant treatment. Conversely, persistent proteinuria/albuminuria indicates the presence of CKD. Persistent proteinuria/albuminuria of renal origin can be defined as positive test results on three or more occasions 2 weeks or longer apart. Because persistent proteinuria/albuminuria can be constant or increase or decrease in magnitude over time, monitoring should use quantitative methods to determine disease trends or response to treatment. Changes in the magnitude of proteinuria should always be interpreted in light of the patient's serum creatinine concentration because proteinuria may decrease in progressive renal disease as the number of functional nephrons decreases. Decreasing proteinuria in the face of stable serum creatinine suggests improving renal function, whereas decreasing proteinuria in the face of increasing serum creatinine suggests disease progression.

IMPLICATIONS OF PROTEINURIA/ALBUMINURIA

In addition to the classic complications of moderate to heavy proteinuria (hypoalbuminemia, edema, ascites, hypercholesterolemia, hypertension, and hypercoagulability), there is increasing evidence in laboratory animals and human beings that proteinuria can cause glomerular and tubulointerstitial damage and result in progressive nephron loss. Proteinuria can arise secondary to immune-mediated, vascular inflammatory, or structural damage to the glomerular capillary wall or as a consequence of intraglomerular hypertension. Plasma proteins that have crossed the glomerular capillary wall can accumulate within the glomerular tuft and stimulate mesangial cell proliferation and increased production of mesangial matrix in human beings [23]. In addition, excessive amounts of protein in the glomerular filtrate can be toxic to human tubular epithelial cells and can lead to interstitial inflammation, fibrosis, and cell death by several mechanisms [24–26]. These mechanisms include tubular obstruction, lysosomal rupture, and complement-mediated and peroxidative damage as well as increased production of cytokines and growth factors.

Several studies in human patients with proteinuric renal disease suggest that proteinuria is associated with renal disease progression. In a study of people with chronic glomerulonephritis, the decrease in proteinuria associated with several different treatments predicted the change in the slope of the reciprocal value of serum creatinine over 6 months [27]. In a 3-year study of 583 human beings with various renal diseases, the angiotensin-converting enzyme (ACE) inhibitor benazepril reduced proteinuria and systemic blood pressure and slowed the decline in glomerular filtration rate (GFR) when compared with placebo treatment [28]. The protective effect of benazepril on renal function was greatest in those patients with substantial proteinuria (>3 g over 24 hours) even after adjustments were made for changes in diastolic blood pressure or urinary protein loss over time [28]. Finally, in a study of 7728 nondiabetic people, overt albuminuria was independently associated with decreased GFR [11].

Evidence linking proteinuria to progression of renal disease in dogs and cats is also beginning to accumulate. In cats with naturally occurring CKD, relatively mild proteinuria (UP/C >0.43) seemed to be negative predictors of survival [29]. In cats with the remnant kidney model of chronic renal failure, proteinuria was associated with nephron hypertrophy, increasing intraglomerular pressures, and hyperfiltration [30]. Interestingly, proteinuria has also been associated with an increased risk of mortality attributable to all causes in cats that have normal renal function when their proteinuria is first detected [31]. In dogs with naturally occurring CKD, the relative risk of uremic crises and mortality was approximately three times greater in dogs with UP/Cs greater than 1.0 (n = 25) compared with dogs with UP/Cs less than 1.0 (n = 20) [32]. In this study, the risk of an adverse outcome was approximately 1.5 times greater for every single-unit increase in UP/C and the decline in renal function was greater in dogs with higher UP/Cs [32]. Individual nephron hyperfiltration and proteinuria have been documented in dogs with the remnant kidney model of renal failure [33]; however, treatments that have slowed the functional decline or histologic changes associated with this model have had variable effects on proteinuria. ACE inhibition and ω-3 fatty acid supplementation have decreased proteinuria and slowed progression [34–36]; however, calcium blockade treatment resulted in increased mesangial cell proliferation despite decreasing proteinuria [34]. Other treatments, such as reduction of dietary phosphorus, decreased renal disease progression in remnant kidney dogs but had no effect on proteinuria. In dogs with experimentally induced immune complex glomerulonephritis, treatment with a thromboxane synthetase inhibitor decreased proteinuria and attenuated the development of glomerular lesions but had no effect on established lesions [37,38]. Reduction of proteinuria by means of an ACE inhibitor (enalapril) was also associated with slowed progression of renal disease in dogs with two different types of naturally occurring glomerulopathies [39,40].

SUMMARY

Proteinuria is a common disorder in dogs and cats that can indicate the presence of CKD before the onset of azotemia or the presence of more severe CKD after the onset of azotemia. Although a direct pathogenetic link between glomerular disease, proteinuria, and progressive renal damage has not been established, attenuation of proteinuria has been associated with decreased renal functional decline in several studies. There is a need to continue to increase our understanding of the effects of proteinuria on the glomerulus, the tubule, and the interstitium in dogs and cats. In addition to being a diagnostic marker of renal disease, proteinuria may also contribute to the progressive nature of canine and feline renal disease. Proteinuria is commonly associated with primary glomerular diseases; however, the loss of renal autoregulation that occurs secondary to nephron loss attributable to any cause (eg, vascular, tubular, interstitial, glomerular) can also result in intraglomerular hypertension and proteinuria. In addition, renal proteinuria can be associated with decreased tubular reabsorption secondary to tubulointerstitial disease.

References

[1] Grauer GF, Moore LE, Smith AR, et al. Comparison of conventional urine protein test strips and a quantitative ELISA for the detection of canine and feline albuminuria. J Vet Intern Med 2004;18:418–9 [abstract].

[2] Vaden SL, Pressler BM, Lappin MR, et al. Urinary tract inflammation has a variable effect on urine albumin concentrations. J Vet Intern Med 2002;16:378 [abstract].

[3] McCaw DL, Knapp DW, Hewett JE. Effect of collection time and exercise restriction on the prevention of urine protein excretion, using urine protein/creatinine ratio in dogs. Am J Vet Res 1985;46:1665–9.

[4] Lees GE, Jensen WA, Simpson DF, et al. Persistent albuminuria precedes onset of overt proteinuria in male dogs with X-linked hereditary nephropathy. J Vet Intern Med 2002;16:353 [abstract].

[5] Lees GE, Brown SA, Elliott J, et al. Assessment and management of proteinuria in dogs and cats; 2004 ACVIM Forum Consensus Statement (small animal). J Vet Intern Med 2005;19: 377–85.

[6] Kruger M, Gordjani N, Burghard R. Post exercise albuminuria in children with different duration of type-1 diabetes mellitus. Pediatr Nephrol 1996;10:594–7.

[7] Hebert LA, Spetie DN, Keane WF. The urgent call of albuminuria/proteinuria: heeding its significance in early detection of kidney disease. Postgrad Med 2001;110:79–96.

[8] Gerstein HC, Mann JF, Yi Q, et al. Albuminuria and risk of cardiovascular events, death, and heart failure in diabetic and nondiabetic individuals. J Am Med Assoc 2001;286: 421–6.

[9] Osterby R, Hartmann A, Nyengaard JR, et al. Development of renal structural lesions in type-1 diabetic patients with microalbuminuria. Observations by light microscopy in 8-year follow-up biopsies. Virchows Arch 2002;440:94–101.

[10] Bakris GL. Microalbuminuria: what is it? Why is it important? What should be done about it? J Clin Hypertens 2001;3:99–102.

[11] Pinto-Sietsma SJ, Janssen WM, Hillege HL, et al. Urinary albumin excretion is associated with renal functional abnormalities in a nondiabetic population. J Am Soc Nephrol 2000;11(10):1882–8.

[12] Keane WF, Eknoyan G. Proteinuria, albuminuria, risk, assessment, detection, elimination (PARADE): a position paper of the National Kidney Foundation. Am J Kidney Dis 1999;33:1004–10.

[13] Grauer GF, Oberhauser EB, Basaraba RJ, et al. Development of microalbuminuria in dogs with heartworm disease. J Vet Intern Med 2002;16:352 [abstract].

[14] Vaden SL, Jensen WA, Longhofer SL, et al. Longitudinal study of microalbuminuria in soft-coated wheaten terriers. J Vet Int Med 2001;15:300 [abstract].

[15] Pressler BM, Vaden SL, Jensen WA. Prevalence of microalbuminuria in dogs evaluated at a referral veterinary hospital. J Vet Intern Med 2001;15:300 [abstract].

[16] Whittemore JC, Jensen WA, Prause L, et al. Comparison of microalbuminuria, urine protein dipstick, and urine protein creatinine ratio results in clinically ill dogs. J Vet Intern Med 2003;17:437 [abstract].

[17] Pressler BM, Proulx DA, Williams LE, et al. Urine albumin concentration is increased in dogs with lymphoma or osteosarcoma. J Vet Intern Med 2003;17:404 [abstract].

[18] Lees GE, Willard MD, Dziezyc J. Glomerular proteinuria is rapidly but reversibly increased by short-term prednisone administration in heterozygous (carrier) female dogs with X-linked hereditary nephropathy. J Vet Intern Med 2002;16:352 [abstract].

[19] Gary AT, Cohn LA, Kerl ME, et al. The effects of exercise on microalbuminuria in dogs. J Vet Intern Med 2003;17:435–6 [abstract].

[20] Grauer GF, Thomas CB, Eicker SW. Estimation of quantitative proteinuria in the dog, using the urine protein-to-creatinine ratio from a random, voided sample. Am J Vet Res 1985;46: 2116–9.

[21] Monroe WE, Davenport DJ, Saunders GK. Twenty-four hour urinary protein loss in healthy cats and the urinary protein to creatinine ratio as an estimate. Am J Vet Res 1989;50: 1906–9.

[22] Adams LG, Polzin DJ, Osborne CA, et al. Correlation of urine protein/creatinine ratio and twenty-four urinary protein excretion in normal cats and cats with induced chronic renal failure. J Vet Intern Med 1992;6:36–40.

[23] Jerums G, Panagiotopoulos S, Tsalamandris C, et al. Why is proteinuria such an important risk factor for progression in clinical trials? Kidney Int 1997;52:S87–92.

[24] Tang S, Sheerin NS, Zhou W, et al. Apical proteins stimulate complement synthesis by cultured human proximal tubular epithelial cells. J Am Soc Nephrol 1999;10:69–76.

[25] Abrass CK. Clinical spectrum and complications of the nephrotic syndrome. J Investig Med 1997;45:143–53.

[26] Eddy A. Role of cellular infiltrates in response to proteinuria. Am J Kidney Dis 2001;37: S25–9.

[27] Gansevoort RT, Navis GJ, Wapstra FH, et al. Proteinuria and progression or renal disease: therapeutic implications. Curr Opin Nephrol Hypertens 1997;6:133–40.

[28] Maschio G, Alberti D, Janin G, et al. Effect of the angiotensin-converting-enzyme inhibitor benazepril on the progression of chronic renal insufficiency. N Engl J Med 1996;334: 939–45.

[29] Syme HM, Elliott J. Relation of survival time and urinary protein excretion in cats with renal failure and/or hypertension. J Vet Intern Med 2003;17:405 [abstract].

[30] Brown SA, Brown CA. Single-nephron adaptations to partial renal ablation in cats. Am J Physiol 1995;269:R1002–8.

[31] Walker D, Syme HM, Markwell P, et al. Predictors of survival in healthy, non-azotemic cats. J Vet Intern Med 2004;18:417 [abstract].

[32] Jacob F, Polzin DJ, Osborne CA, et al. Evaluation of the association between initial proteinuria and morbidity rate or death in dogs with naturally occurring chronic renal failure. J Am Vet Med Assoc 2005;226:393–400.

[33] Brown SA, Finco DR, Crowell WA, et al. Single-nephron adaptation to partial renal ablation in the dog. Am J Physiol 1990;258:F495–503.

[34] Brown SA, Walton CL, Crawford P, et al. Long-term effects of antihypertensive regimens on renal hemodynamics and proteinuria. Kidney Int 1993;43:1210–8.

[35] Brown SA, Brown CA, Crowell WA, et al. Beneficial effects of chronic administration of dietary ω-3 polyunsaturated fatty acids in dogs with renal insufficiency. J Lab Clin Med 1998;131:447–55.

[36] Brown SA, Finco DR, Brown CA, et al. Evaluation of the effects of inhibition of angiotensin converting enzyme with enalapril in dogs with induced chronic renal insufficiency. Am J Vet Res 2003;64:321–7.

[37] Longhofer SL, Frisbie DD, Johnson HC, et al. Effects of thromboxane synthetase inhibition on immune complex glomerulonephritis. Am J Vet Res 1991;52:480–7.

[38] Grauer GF, Frisbie DD, Longhofer SL, et al. Effects of a thromboxane synthetase inhibitor on established immune complex glomerulonephritis in dogs. Am J Vet Res 1992;53:808–13.

[39] Grodecki KM, Gains MJ, Baumal R, et al. Treatment of X-linked hereditary nephritis in Samoyed dogs with angiotensin converting enzyme (ACE) inhibitor. J Comp Pathol 1997;117: 209–25.

[40] Grauer GF, Greco DS, Getzy DM, et al. Effects of enalapril vs placebo as a treatment for canine idiopathic glomerulonephritis. J Vet Intern Med 2000;14:526–33.

Interpretation of Liver Enzymes

Sharon A. Center, DVM

Department of Clinical Sciences, College of Veterinary Medicine,
Cornell University, Ithaca, NY 14853, USA

Biochemical screening tests facilitated by convenient automated chemical analyses are commonly used for routine health assessments. The presence of liver disease is often first recognized on the basis of liver enzymes. Although liver enzyme measurements are sometimes referred to as "liver function tests," they reflect hepatocyte membrane integrity, hepatocyte or biliary epithelial necrosis, cholestasis, or induction phenomenon rather than liver functional capacity. Interpretation of liver enzymes must be integrated with consideration of the patient's database, including the medical history, physical examination findings, other routine laboratory test results, specific assessments of liver function, and imaging studies. Confirmation of a specific liver disease usually requires acquisition of a liver biopsy. This article provides a clinical review of the most commonly used liver enzymes in small animal practice.

INITIAL PATTERN RECOGNITION

In a general patient population, abnormally increased liver enzyme activity is considerably more common than the prevalence of liver disease. This relates to the influence of systemic disorders on the liver. Occupying a sentinel position between the alimentary canal and systemic circulatory system, the liver has wide exposure to toxins and drug metabolites, endotoxins, and infectious agents. Consequently, a wide spectrum of nonhepatic disorders may influence liver enzyme activity.

The pattern of liver enzyme abnormalities in relation to the signalment, history, total bilirubin concentration, serum bile acid values, and comorbid conditions or medications provides the first indication of a liver-specific disorder. The full assessment of the liver enzyme aberration takes into consideration (1) the predominant pattern of enzyme change (hepatocellular leakage enzymes versus cholestatic enzymes), (2) the fold increase of enzyme activity greater than the normal reference range (using arbitrary cutoffs, the magnitudes of increased enzyme activity are considered as mild, <5 times the upper reference range; moderate, 5–10 times the upper reference range; or marked, >10 times

E-mail address: sac6@cornell.edu

0195-5616/07/$ – see front matter
doi:10.1016/j.cvsm.2006.11.009

the upper reference range), (3) the rate of change (increase or resolution), and (4) the nature of the course of change (fluctuation versus progressive increase or decrement). The reference range reflects the mean value within 2 standard deviations observed in a "normal" population. Thus, up to 2.5% of normal individuals can have borderline abnormal enzyme values. The specificities (number of negative tests in individuals lacking the disease of interest) of the most commonly used serum enzymes in dogs and cats are summarized in Fig. 1, as taken from a population of dogs (n = 915) and cats (n = 534) with biopsy-confirmed liver status. These animals (100 dogs and 66 cats) were initially suspected of having liver disease but were proven not to have liver disease on the basis of liver biopsy.

Recognizing whether enzyme abnormalities are persistent or cyclic helps to categorize different hepatobiliary disorders. For example, dogs and cats with nonsuppurative necroinflammatory hepatitis or cholangitis may have widely fluctuating liver enzymes in the absence of overt illness in the early stages of the syndrome. Animals exposed to toxins causing hepatic necrosis may have astounding transaminase activity that dissipates over time. Investigating liver function with paired fasting and postprandial serum bile acid determinations or urine bile acid or creatinine measurements (urine collected 4–8 hours after meal ingestion) may expedite pursuit of a liver biopsy when clinical signs remain vague and serum liver enzymes are only mildly increased. Finding high bile acid values corroborates the need for histologic investigations. Imaging studies, including thoracic and abdominal radiographs, assist in detecting primary underlying disorders that have secondarily influenced the liver (causing increased release of liver enzymes). Ultrasonographic interrogation of the

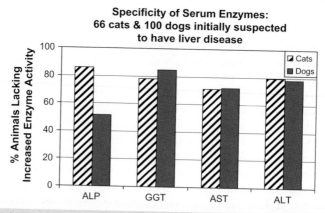

Fig. 1. Specificity of routinely used serum enzymes applied as screening tests in health surveillance of dogs and cats. Data represent the percentage of animals lacking liver disease (liver biopsy completed) having a negative test result. Additional data from this large clinical population are provided in other figures in this article. ALP, alkaline phosphatase; ALT, alanine aminotransferase; AST, aspartate aminotransferase; GGT, γ-glutamyltransferase. (*Data from* the New York State College of Veterinary Medicine, Cornell University, Ithaca, NY, 2006.)

hepatobiliary system helps to identify focal abnormalities, involvement of biliary structures, perfusion abnormalities, and general changes in hepatic parenchymal echogenicity. Thoracic radiographs assist in the recognition of metastatic lesions, primary cardiopulmonary disease, and presence of an enlarged sternal lymph node reflecting abdominal disease (eg, inflammation, neoplasia).

Diagnostic enzymology involves the interpretation of serum enzymes originally located within the hepatocyte or attached to its plasma membrane. The process of enzyme release may be as simple as altered membrane integrity (direct efflux to the sinusoidal compartment through leaky gap junctions), cell necrosis, release of membrane-bound enzymes with membrane fragments (in necrotizing, metastatic, infiltrative, and cholestatic liver disorders), or release of membrane-bound enzymes from their phosphatidylinositol anchor as soluble fractions [1]. A general overview of the enzymes discussed in this article is provided in Table 1.

AMINOTRANSFERASES: ALANINE AMINOTRANSFERASE AND ASPARTATE AMINOTRANSFERASE

The serum aminotransferases (aspartate aminotransferase [AST], previously called serum glutamate-oxaloacetate aminotransferase [SGOT], and alanine aminotransferase [ALT], previously called serum glutamate-pyruvate aminotransferase [SGPT]), are commonly measured as a means of detecting liver injury. These enzymes catalyze the transfer of the α-amino groups of aspartate and alanine to the α-keto group of α-ketoglutaric acid (α-KG), which are reactions essential for gluconeogenesis and urea formation (Fig. 2).

ALT facilitates the mobilization of carbon and nitrogen from muscle (in the form of alanine) to the liver, where it can be used for protein synthesis, energy production, and nitrogen elimination in the urea cycle. In the liver, ALT transfers ammonia to α-KG, regenerating pyruvate that can be diverted for gluconeogenesis. Overall, this process is referred to as the glucose-alanine cycle (Fig. 3).

ALT and AST are present in high concentrations in liver but also exist in other tissues (Figs. 4 and 5) [2,3]. AST is present not only in the liver but in higher concentrations in the kidney, heart, and skeletal muscle and in measurable amounts in the brain, small intestine, and spleen. Comparatively, ALT is primarily located in the liver, with concentrations 4-fold higher than in the next most abundant site (cardiac muscle) and 10-fold higher than in the kidney. In health, the hepatocellular ALT activity is 10,000-fold greater than in plasma. Distribution of ALT and AST within the hepatocyte is variable (Fig. 6). Although most transaminases reside within the soluble fraction of the cytosol, an important component of AST resides within mitochondria (20%) [4]. The distribution of transaminases within the acinar zones also differs. ALT achieves higher concentrations in periportal hepatocytes, and AST achieves higher concentrations in periacinar (zone 3) hepatocytes. Consequently, the relative activity of ALT or AST in serum may reflect the acinar zone of liver injury [5].

Table 1
Liver enzymes

Cytosolic enzymes	ALT	Primarily located in hepatocyte cytosol, with higher values in periportal cells (zone 1) Rapidly leaks with altered membrane integrity and persists for days $t_{1/2}$ controversial, ranging from hours to many days, removed by sinusoidal hepatocytes, removal may be impaired in severe liver disease augmenting high enzymes
	LDH	Wide tissue distribution, with highest concentrations (in descending order) in skeletal muscle, heart, and kidney, with lesser amounts in intestine, liver, lung, and pancreas Multiple isozymes: LDH_5 predominates in liver and contributes to serum LDH Poor specificity because biochemistry profiles report total LDH High LDH activity in diffuse severe hepatic necrosis or inflammation, myositis, muscle trauma, and lymphosarcoma external to liver Rapid $t_{1/2}$, transiently increases only during active necrosis
	SDH	Released during hepatic degeneration or necrosis or secondarily to altered membrane permeability Highest tissue concentrations in liver Reflects ongoing hepatocellular injury but offers no advantage over ALT In vitro lability during transport complicates interpretation
Cytosolic or mitochondrial	AST	Present in multiple tissues, including skeletal muscle, cardiac muscle, kidney, brain, and liver Located in hepatocyte cytosol (80%) and mitochondria (20%) Rapidly leaks with altered membrane integrity Prominence in zone 3 Mitochondrial enzyme leaks in necrosis AST may have higher sensitivity for liver injury in some animals compared with ALT $t_{1/2}$ controversial, ranging from minutes to hours in dog, 77 minutes in cat
	Arginase	Exclusive to liver, located in hepatocyte cytosol and mitochondria Rapidly leaks with substantial membrane injury Modest increases with glucocorticoid induction in dogs $t_{1/2}$ short, such that it only marks acute severe tissue damage

(continued on next page)

Table 1 (continued)		
Membrane-bound enzymes	ALP	Multiple isoenzymes, isozymes, or isoforms
		Liver-, bone-, intestinal-, placental-, and glucocorticoid-induced (latter in dogs only)
		Liver-induced ALP in biliary membranes, glucocorticoid-induced ALP in sinusoidal hepatocyte membranes
		Isoenzyme characterization has limited clinical value
		Bone-induced ALP is increased in juvenile animals with bone growth, hyperthyroid cats, and bone inflammation or neoplasia
		Liver-induced ALP and glucocorticoid-induced ALP undergo induction phenomenon in dogs glucocorticoid-induced ALP associated with acquired glycogen vacuolar hepatopathy (in dogs)
		Canine ALP $t_{1/2}$ liver-induced ALP = 70 hours, glucocorticoid-induced ALP = 70 hours, intestinal-induced ALP = 6 minutes
		Feline ALP $t_{1/2}$ liver-induced ALP = 6 hours, intestinal-induced ALP <2 minutes
	γ-GT	Present in multiple tissues, kidney, pancreas, intestine, and liver
		Liver γ-GT is a major source of serum enzyme
		Biliary membrane localization: highest values in cholestatic disorders
		Glucocorticoid γ-GT induction in dogs
		$t_{1/2}$ not determined in dogs or cats

Abbreviations: ALP, alkaline phosphatase; AST, aspartate aminotransferase; γ-GT, γ-glutamyltransferase; $t_{1/2}$, half-life.

The location of transaminases in the soluble cytosolic fraction of the hepatocyte allows immediate release with even minor changes in hepatocellular membrane permeability. This indiscriminant transaminase leakage limits the diagnostic value of these enzymes for differentiating reversible or irreversible membrane changes as well as the extent of tissue involvement. Nevertheless, the magnitude of transaminase activity does seem to correlate with the number of involved cells. Transaminases leak into the perisinusoidal space from the sinusoidal borders of hepatocytes or through leaky gap junctions into the ultrafiltrate in the space of Disse. From here, they diffuse through the dynamic fenestrae in the sinusoidal endothelium and mingle with the systemic circulation.

Hepatic transaminases are known to increase with muscle injury as well as after vigorous physical activity in dogs [6]. Regarding exercise, it remains unclear whether these enzymes "escape" from hepatocytes or originate from well-perfused active muscle [7,8]. A 1.4- to 2-fold increase in plasma AST associated with increases in creatine kinase (CK) and lactate dehydrogenase (LDH) has been shown in dogs after moderate to severe short-term exercise

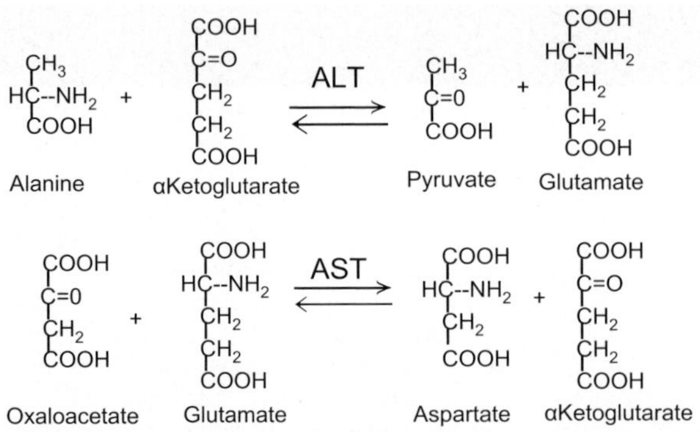

$$
\begin{array}{ccc}
\text{Alanine} & \alpha\text{Ketoglutarate} & \xrightarrow{\text{ALT}} & \text{Pyruvate} & \text{Glutamate}
\end{array}
$$

$$
\begin{array}{ccc}
\text{Oxaloacetate} & \text{Glutamate} & \xrightarrow{\text{AST}} & \text{Aspartate} & \alpha\text{Ketoglutarate}
\end{array}
$$

Fig. 2. Reactions catalyzed by the aminotransferases commonly measured as markers of hepatocellular injury.

(15-minute run at 16 km/h with a 10% incline). Similarly, a 1.4- to 2.9-fold increase in plasma AST and lactic dehydrogenase occurred in dogs after electrophysiologic stimulation of hind limb muscles (10 pulses per second for 30 minutes) [9].

The half-life ($t_{1/2}$) of transaminases remains controversial, with estimates ranging between 3 hours and 17 days made using intravenous injections of hepatic homogenates [3,10]. In one study, three dogs injected with a 20% liver tissue homogenate (sampled over 70 hours) demonstrated an average $t_{1/2}$ for AST of 263 minutes and for ALT of 149 minutes [3]. Another study (15,000-g liver homogenate supernatant [ALT = 254 U/g and AST = 382 U/g] given intravenously to seven dogs) demonstrated sustained plasma transaminase elevations for 13 to 17 days for ALT and for 3 to 5 days for AST [10]. A $t_{1/2}$ for ALT of 59 ± 9 hours and for AST of 22 ± 1.6 hours was calculated

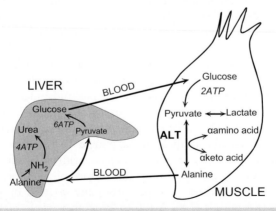

Fig. 3. Drawing depicts the function of ALT in the glucose-alanine cycle, as described in the text.

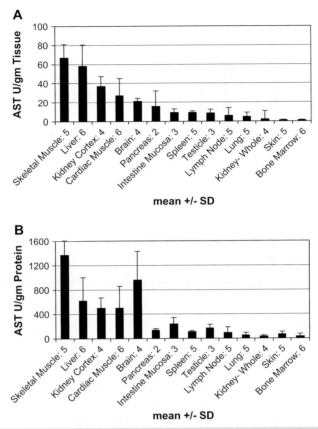

Fig. 4. Tissue distribution of AST in dogs on the basis of units of activity per wet tissue weight (*A*) and per tissue protein concentration (*B*). Numbers affiliated with the tissue label indicate the number of dogs sampled. (*Data from* Nagode LA, Frajola WJ, Loeb WF. Enzyme activities of canine tissues. Am J Vet Res 1966;27:1385–93.)

[10]. The plasma $t_{1/2}$ of AST in the cat has been estimated to be 77 minutes [11]. Considering that it requires five times the $t_{1/2}$ for plasma clearance, long-term persistence of transaminases may contribute to sustained high serum enzyme activities in some disorders. Because catabolism of transaminases occurs by absorptive endocytosis in the sinusoidal hepatocytes, slow enzyme clearance may augment high plasma enzyme activity in patients with substantial liver disease (eg, acquired portosystemic shunting, nodular regeneration, hepatic fibrosis) [12,13].

Alanine Aminotransferase

The largest increases in ALT develop with hepatocellular necrosis and inflammation. In this circumstance, gradual and sequential decreases in ALT activity can be a sign of recovery. In acute liver disease, a 50% or more decrease in serum ALT activity over several days is considered a good prognostic sign.

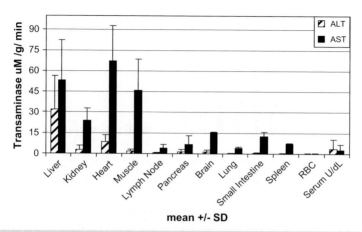

Fig. 5. Comparative tissue distribution of AST and ALT in dogs (n = 6) on the basis of micromoles per gram wet liver tissue weight per minute. (*Data from* Zinkl JG, Bush RM, Cornelius CE, et al. Comparative studies on plasma and tissue sorbitol, glutamic, lactic, and hydroxybutyric dehydrogenase and transaminase activities in the dog. Res Vet Sci 1971;12:211–14.)

Some animals with severe disease have normal serum ALT activity, however. It is also important to acknowledge that declining serum ALT activity may represent a paucity of viable hepatocytes in chronic liver disease or severe toxicity or even toxin-suppressed transaminase synthesis (eg, microcystin, aflatoxin).

After acute severe hepatocellular necrosis, serum ALT activity usually increases markedly and sharply within 24 to 48 hours to values greater than or equal to 100-fold normal, peaking during the first 5 postinjury days [14–20]. If the injurious event resolves, ALT activity gradually declines to normal over a 2- to 3-week interval. Although this pattern is considered "classic," some severe hepatotoxins are not associated with profound or protracted serum transaminase activity. This is encountered with toxins that inhibit transaminase

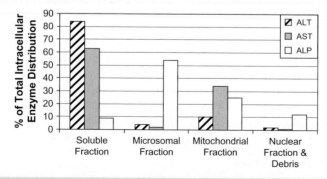

Fig. 6. Distribution of ALT, AST, and alkaline phosphatase (ALP) in the canine liver. (*Adapted from* Keller P. Enzyme activities in the dog: tissue analyses, plasma values, and intracellular distribution. Am J Vet Res 1981;41:575–82.)

gene transcription or that otherwise interfere with transaminase biosynthesis (eg, aflatoxin B_1 hepatotoxicity, microcystin hepatotoxicity) [21,22].

Classic toxins used to exemplify the clinical response to a necrotizing hepatotoxin are carbon tetrachloride (CCl_4^-), acetaminophen, and nitrosamine. Data from experimentally intoxicated patients were used to exemplify enzymatic response patterns. Hepatocellular necrosis induced by nitrosamines increases plasma ALT activity, but this increase was not significant until after 1 week of intermittent chronic exposure. The increase in transaminase activity persists for weeks until the necrosis resolves. Low-grade hepatocellular degeneration is also observed in some dogs with portosystemic shunts (PSSs). Released enzymes in these patients may have delayed sinusoidal clearance because histologic changes are minor. Changes in plasma ALT activity before and after exposure of dogs to nitrosamines, before and after surgical creation of PSSs, and in a clinical patient that survived food-borne aflatoxin hepatotoxicity are profiled in Fig. 7. This figure exemplifies the influence of different forms of liver injury on serum enzyme profiles [20,23]. Hepatotoxicity induced by acetaminophen is the classic example of hepatotoxicity induced by an electrophile adduct. Marked increases in plasma ALT and AST activities develop within 24 hours, yet these may decline within 72 hours to near-normal values. This toxin is highly dose dependent in dogs and cats. The ALT profiles in animals receiving nonlethal and lethal amounts of acetaminophen are illustrated in Fig. 8 [24–28]. Cats are exceedingly susceptible to acetaminophen toxicosis, with hematologic signs dominating their clinical presentation after as little as 125 mg. Although dogs are more resistant than cats, a dose of 200 mg/kg of body weight may be life endangering.

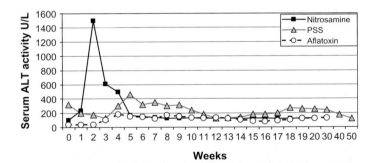

Fig. 7. Plasma ALT activity profiles before and after short-term exposure of dogs to nitrosamines, before and after surgical creation of PSSs that produced low-grade hepatic degeneration, and in a clinical patient that survived severe food-borne aflatoxin hepatotoxicity. (*Data from* the New York State College of Veterinary Medicine, Cornell University, Ithaca, NY, 2006; Strombeck DR, Harrold D, Rogers Q, et al. Plasma amino acids, glucagon, and insulin concentrations in dogs with nitrosamine-induced hepatic disease. Am J Vet Res 1983;44: 2028–2036; and Schaeffer MC, Rogers QR, Buffington CA, et al. Long-term biochemical and physiologic effects of surgically placed portacaval shunts in dogs. Am J Vet Res 1986;47:346–55.)

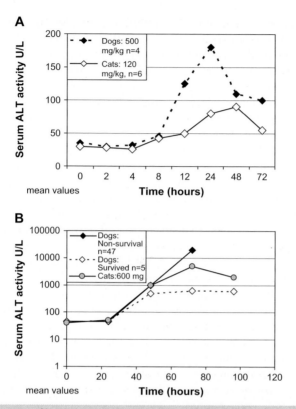

Fig. 8. Plasma ALT profiles in dogs and cats receiving nonlethal (*A*) and lethal (*B*) amounts of acetaminophen. (*Data from* references 24–27).

Acute hepatic necrosis caused by infectious canine hepatitis (adenovirus) increases plasma ALT activity by 30-fold, with enzyme activity peaking within 4 days [29]. Thereafter, a chronic sustained increase in ALT is common, and the patient may develop chronic hepatitis. This infectious disorder is now rarely encountered in companion dogs in North America. Hepatic injury induced by toxins usually causes plasma ALT activity to increase, peak, and normalize sooner than observed in infectious viral hepatitis. Chronic hepatitis, a persistent necroinflammatory disorder, is associated with varying severities of necrosis and fibrosis, cyclic disease activity, and plasma enzyme "flares." At times, plasma ALT activity achieves values 10-fold normal or greater. Enzyme fluctuations contrast with enzyme profiles associated with a single injurious event or toxin exposure. In these latter cases, serum ALT activity declines as injury resolves, but serum ALP activity may increase as a result of the regenerative proliferative process. The sensitivity of ALT in the detection of hepatobiliary syndromes in the dog and cat is shown in Fig. 9 using clinical data from 815

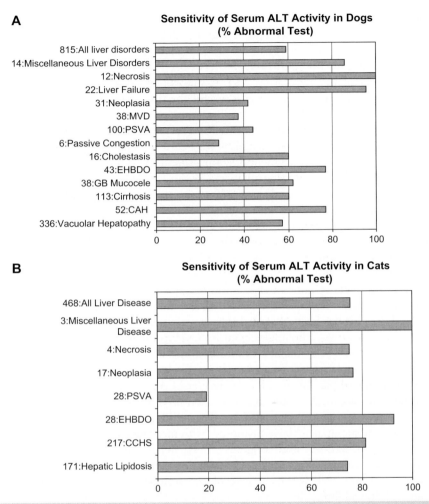

Fig. 9. Sensitivity of serum ALT activity for the detection of hepatobiliary syndromes in the dog (A) and cat (B). The number preceding the disease description indicates the number of cases included. Miscellaneous liver disorders included syndromes that could not be classified in other categories and for which there were fewer than five cases. CAH, chronic "active" hepatitis; CCHS, cholangitis or cholangiohepatitis syndrome of cats; EHBDO, extrahepatic bile duct occlusion; GB, gallbladder; MVD, microvascular dysplasia; PSVA, portosystemic vascular anomaly. All diagnoses were confirmed by liver biopsy or definitive imaging studies in dogs with a PSVA. (*Data from* the New York State College of Veterinary Medicine, Cornell University, Ithaca, NY, 2006.)

dogs and 468 cats with biopsy-confirmed disorders. Unfortunately, the high sensitivity of ALT in some disorders is not linked to high specificity for differentiating clinically significant liver disease or specific histologic abnormalities or for identifying dogs with hepatic dysfunction.

Aspartate Aminotransferase

As previously discussed (see Figs. 4 and 5), AST is present in substantial concentrations in a wide variety of tissues [2,3,11,14,30]. Distinct hepatocellular cytosolic and mitochondrial isozymes have been proven in several species. In people, most of the circulating AST is mitochondrial in origin, and the extremely short $t_{1/2}$ of this isozyme is useful for distinguishing severe ongoing hepatocellular insult [31].

Increased serum AST activity can reflect reversible or irreversible changes in hepatocellular membrane permeability, cell necrosis, hepatic inflammation, and, in the dog, microsomal enzyme induction. After acute diffuse severe hepatic necrosis, serum AST activity sharply increases during the first 3 days to values 10- to 30-fold normal in dogs and up to 50-fold normal in cats [14,16,32]. If necrosis resolves, the serum AST activity gradually declines over 2 to 3 weeks. In most cases, AST activity generally parallels changes in ALT activity. In some animals, however, AST becomes quiescent before ALT [14]. Although increased AST activity in the absence of abnormal ALT activity implicates an extrahepatic enzyme source (notably muscle injury), there are clinical exceptions that may relate to the severity and zonal location of hepatic damage. In some cats with liver disease, AST performs as a more sensitive marker of liver injury compared with ALT. This has been observed in cats with a variety of syndromes, including hepatic necrosis, cholangiohepatitis, myeloproliferative disease and lymphoma associated with hepatic infiltration, and chronic bile duct obstruction. This trend is evident by comparing sensitivities for ALT and AST, as displayed in Figs. 9 and 10 [32,33]. A similar behavior of AST noted in fewer dogs with naturally developing liver disease is corroborated by conclusions made in two retrospective studies of canine liver disease [34,35]. Contribution of AST from other tissues, particularly in animals with metastatic neoplasia, systemic inflammatory conditions, and congestive heart failure, may help to explain enzyme performance. Dogs treated with glucocorticoids may develop mildly increased serum AST activity that resolves within several weeks of glucocorticoid withdrawal [36].

ALKALINE PHOSPHATASE

Alkaline phosphatase (ALP) is a member of a family of zinc metalloprotein enzymes that split terminal phosphate groups from organic phosphate esters. These enzymes function at membranous interfaces and operate best at an alkaline pH. The exact functions of ALP in intermediary metabolism continue to be refined. Unlike transaminases, ALP is attached to cell membranes by glucosyl phosphatidylinositol linkages. These "anchors" must be cleaved by endogenous phospholipases before soluble enzyme can be distributed into the systemic circulation [37–39]. Release of ALP from its membrane linkage is facilitated in the presence of bile acids that exert a detergent-like influence on the membrane anchor; this action also augments ALP release in cholestatic disorders [37,38]. Increased serum ALP activity in the dog is the most common biochemical abnormality on routine biochemical profiles. It is also a biochemical test that

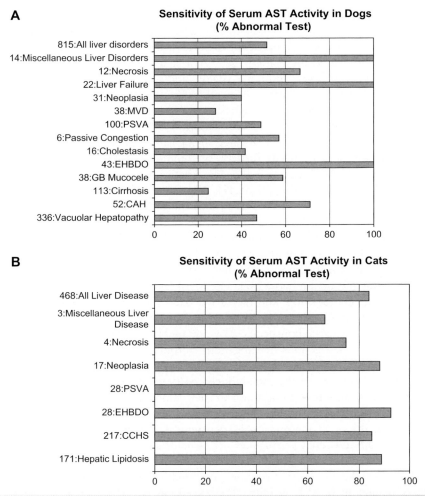

Fig. 10. Sensitivity of serum AST activity for the detection of hepatobiliary syndromes in the dog (*A*) and cat (*B*). The number preceding the disease description indicates the number of cases included. Miscellaneous liver disorders included syndromes that could not be classified in other categories and for which there were fewer than five cases. CAH, chronic "active" hepatitis; CCHS, cholangitis or cholangiohepatitis syndrome of cats; EHBDO, extrahepatic bile duct occlusion; GB, gallbladder; MVD, microvascular dysplasia; PSVA, portosystemic vascular anomaly. All diagnoses were confirmed by liver biopsy or definitive imaging studies in dogs with a PSVA. (*Data from* the New York State College of Veterinary Medicine, Cornell University, Ithaca, NY, 2006.)

can defy diagnostic scrutiny in the dog, with ALP having the lowest specificity of the routinely used liver enzymes (see Fig. 1). The diagnostic complexity involving this enzyme in the dog involves the regulation and induction phenomenon that influence ALP isozyme gene transcription.

Tissues containing the highest quantities of ALP in the dog, in descending order, are the intestinal mucosa, kidney (cortex), placenta, liver, and bone. Tissue concentrations of ALP in cats have been variably reported: Hoffmann and colleagues [40] found the highest tissue ALP activity in the intestine, followed by the renal cortex, liver, and bone. Everett and colleagues [41] found the highest ALP activity in the kidney, followed by the intestine, bone, and liver, and Foster and Thoday [42] found highest concentrations in the kidney, followed by the intestine, liver, and bone. Distinct serum ALP isozymes can be extracted from some of these tissues. The three major isozymes encountered in canine serum include bone-induced (B-ALP), liver-induced (L-ALP), and glucocorticoid-induced (G-ALP) enzymes [43–46]. There are two genes responsible for ALP production in the dog [37,38,47]. The first is the tissue-nonspecific ALP gene that transcribes L-ALP, B-ALP, and the kidney-induced ALP isoforms (isoforms are similar forms of an enzyme transcribed from the same gene but having different posttranslational processing) [37]. These ALP isoforms differ only in their degree of glycosylation. The second gene, the intestinal ALP gene, is specific for the intestinal-induced ALP isoenzyme product (I-ALP) produced in the intestinal mucosa [37]. The I-ALP and G-ALP forms differ only in carbohydrate composition, and recent work has confirmed that G-ALP is synthesized in the liver, where it is attached to perisinusoidal membranes of hepatocytes [37]. The tissue-nonspecific ALP and G-ALP can be induced in dogs but not in cats by endogenous or exogenous steroidogenic hormones and certain drugs.

In dogs, the $t_{1/2}$ of the placental-induced ALP, renal-induced ALP, and I-ALP are short (<6 minutes). In addition to their short $t_{1/2}$, intestinal and renal isozymes are excreted into the intestinal lumen and urine, respectively [43,48]. In the cat, the $t_{1/2}$ of the intestinal isoenzyme is less than 2 minutes. Because the placental and renal isoenzymes are structurally similar, they are also surmised to have a short $t_{1/2}$ in the systemic circulation [40,47,49]. The isozymes with an ultrashort $t_{1/2}$ are not routinely detected in canine or feline serum in patients having high ALP activity. The exception is the placental isoenzyme, which has been detected in late-term pregnant cats [49]. In dogs, L-ALP and G-ALP are primarily responsible for high serum ALP activity, whereas L-ALP is primarily responsible in the cat. Juvenile dogs and cats maintain higher serum ALP activity than mature adult animals, however, as a result of higher bone metabolism and B-ALP release associated with bone growth and remodeling [40,43,49,50]. The $t_{1/2}$ of L-ALP and G-ALP in the dog is approximately 70 hours [43,46,48], whereas the $t_{1/2}$ of L-ALP in the cat is remarkably shorter at approximately 6 hours [40,47,49]. Increased total serum ALP activity develops in 43% to 75% of hyperthyroid cats, depending on the chronicity of their endocrinopathy [51,52]. The B-ALP isoenzyme may substantially contribute to the total ALP activity in these cats, similar to hyperthyroid human beings (Fig. 11) [42,50,53–58]. Evidence of enhanced bone mobilization (increased osteocalcin), increased parathormone, and reduced ionized calcium has been demonstrated in hyperthyroid cats with high serum ALP activity. Further, in

A

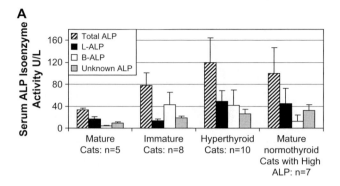

B

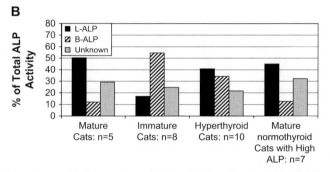

Fig. 11. Serum ALP isoenzyme activity in mature and immature healthy cats, hyperthyroid cats, and mature euthyroid cats with high serum ALP activity (A) and the percentage of total ALP activity in each group (B). (*Data from* Horney BS, Farmer AJ, Honor DJ, et al. Agarose gel electrophoresis of alkaline phosphatase isoenzymes in the serum of hyperthyroid cats. Vet Clin Pathol, 1994:23:98–102.)

one study, 88% of cats had measurable serum L-ALP and B-ALP isozymes whether or not they had high serum ALP activity [42].

The comparably small magnitudes of ALP activity in cats with liver disease (twofold to threefold normal) relative to the dog (often >fourfold to fivefold normal) reflect the lower specific activity of hepatic ALP in cats and the shorter L-ALP enzyme $t_{1/2}$ [11,49]. Nevertheless, this difference does not diminish the clinical utility of serum ALP in the diagnosis of feline liver disease when the species-appropriate perspective is maintained (see Fig. 1; Figs. 12 and 13).

The utility of serum ALP activity as a diagnostic indicator in the dog is complicated by the common accumulation of the L-ALP and G-ALP isozymes. Studies confirm that the canine liver is the common site of L-ALP and G-ALP synthesis in response to steroidogenic hormones [59,60]. The clinical utility of ALP in the dog is not improved by differentiating ALP isoenzymes, because the G-ALP isoenzyme is so easily induced by chronic stress and perhaps inflammatory mediators associated with systemic disease and spontaneous liver disorders. Glucocorticoid exposure imparts a rapid but transient increase in L-ALP

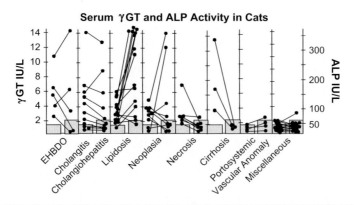

Fig. 12. Dot-plot shows serum ALP and γ-glutamyltransferase (γ-GT) activity in cats with biopsy-confirmed spontaneous hepatobiliary disorders. Miscellaneous represents cats with nonhepatobiliary disorders. Boxes in lanes represent the reference range. EHBDO, extrahepatic bile duct occlusion. (*Data from* the New York State College of Veterinary Medicine, Cornell University, Ithaca, NY.)

induction or production that plateaus within 7 to 10 days. In contrast, the G-ALP undergoes an initial 10-day transcription lag phase; this phenomenon is shown in Fig. 14 [59].

The B-ALP isozyme increases secondary to osteoblast activity. This isozyme is detected, as previously mentioned, in the serum of young growing animals and may also be detected in patients with bone tumors, secondary renal hyperparathyroidism, or osteomyelitis. The contribution of B-ALP to the total serum ALP activity usually does not lead to an erroneous diagnosis of cholestatic liver disease, however [43]. Bone remodeling secondary to neoplasia may not substantially affect serum ALP activity or may cause only a trivial two- to threefold increase in the dog. In the young growing cat, however, increased serum B-ALP activity may simulate enzyme activity realized with hepatobiliary disease.

The L-ALP isozyme is derived from membranes in the canalicular area of the hepatocyte and refluxes into plasma secondary to enhanced de novo hepatic synthesis, canalicular injury, cholestasis, and solubilization of membrane-bound protein by the detergent action of bile salts [43,61–66].

Although ALT is immediately released from the hepatocellular cytosol in acute hepatic necrosis, the small quantities of membrane-bound ALP cannot be readily dispatched. Rather, it takes several days for induction of membrane-associated enzyme to "gear up" and spill into the perisinusoidal ultrafiltrate in the space of Disse. The liver ramps up L-ALP production at a faster rate than G-ALP, even in the presence of glucocorticoids. The L-ALP rapidly plateaus, however; thereafter, the G-ALP assumes a dominant role in total serum ALP activity in patients with chronically increased enzyme activity. The largest increases in serum ALP activity (L-ALP or G-ALP 100-fold normal or greater) develop in dogs with diffuse or focal cholestatic disorders, massive

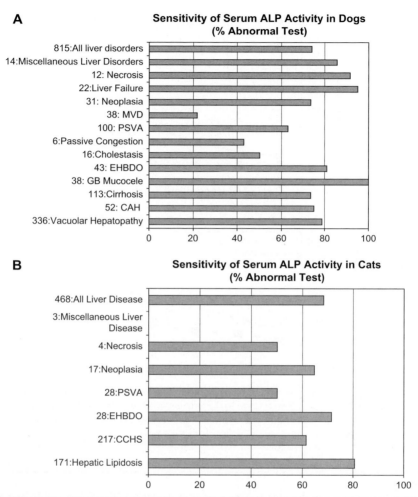

Fig. 13. Sensitivity of serum ALP activity for the detection of hepatobiliary syndromes in the dog (A) and cat (B). The number preceding the disease description indicates the number of cases included. Miscellaneous liver disorders included disorders that could not be classified in other categories and for which there were fewer than five cases. CAH, chronic "active" hepatitis; CCHS, cholangitis or cholangiohepatitis syndrome of cats; EHBDO, extrahepatic bile duct occlusion; GB, gallbladder; MVD, microvascular dysplasia; PSVA, portosystemic vascular anomaly. All diagnoses were confirmed by liver biopsy or definitive imaging studies in dogs with a PSVA. (*Data from* the New York State College of Veterinary Medicine, Cornell University, Ithaca, NY, 2006.)

hepatocellular carcinoma (HCCA), or bile duct carcinoma and in those treated with glucocorticoids.

Although serum activity of ALP may be normal or only modestly increased in dogs with metastatic neoplasia involving the liver, a dramatic increase in serum ALP may be realized in dogs with mammary neoplasia. Approximately

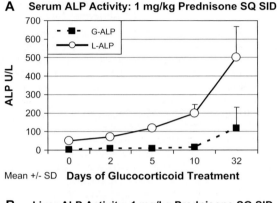

A **Serum ALP Activity: 1 mg/kg Prednisone SQ SID**

Mean +/- SD **Days of Glucocorticoid Treatment**

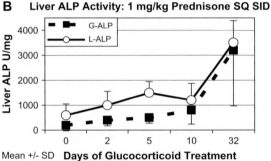

B **Liver ALP Activity: 1 mg/kg Prednisone SQ SID**

Mean +/- SD **Days of Glucocorticoid Treatment**

Fig. 14. Sequential measurements of L-ALP and G-ALP isoenzymes in dogs before and after initiation of prednisolone at a dose of 1 mg/kg administered subcutaneously (SQ) once daily (SID). Data depict the acute initial rise in serum L-ALP activity and the later increase in liver tissue L-ALP. (*Data from* Wiedmeyer CE, Solter PE, Hoffmann WE. Kinetics of mRNA expression of alkaline phosphatase isoenzymes in hepatic tissues from glucocorticoid-treated dogs. Am J Vet Res. 2002;63:1089–95.)

55% of dogs with malignant mammary tumors and 47% of dogs with benign mammary tumors develop high serum ALP activity [67,68]. Although there was no significant difference in total ALP activity between dogs with malignant and benign neoplasms (with and without osseous transformations), the highest serum ALP activity developed in dogs with malignant mixed tumors. This association has not been reconciled with osseous transformation or myoepithelial ALP production within tumor tissue. Approximately 11% of dogs with malignant tumors and 7% of dogs with benign tumors developed a fourfold increase in serum ALP activity. Nevertheless, serum ALP has no value as a diagnostic or prognostic marker in dogs with mammary neoplasia. It remains unclear whether disease remission (eg, treatment involving surgery or chemotherapy) is followed by a regression in serum ALP activity and whether serum ALP activity functions as a paraneoplastic marker of mammary neoplasia.

After acute severe hepatic necrosis, ALP activity increases two- to fivefold normal (in the dog and cat), stabilizes, and then gradually declines over 2 to

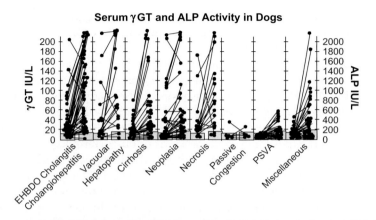

Fig. 15. Dot-plot shows serum ALP and γ-glutamyltransferase (γ-GT) activity in 270 dogs with biopsy-confirmed spontaneous hepatobiliary disorders. Miscellaneous represents dogs with nonhepatobiliary disorders. Boxes in lane represent the reference range. EHBDO, extrahepatic bile duct obstruction; PSVA, portosystemic vascular anoma. (*Data from* the New York State College of Veterinary Medicine, Cornell University, Ithaca, NY.)

3 weeks [18,69]. Sustained ALP activity often reconciles with biliary epithelial hyperplasia associated with the proliferative reparative process that follows panlobular necrosis. Thereafter, ALP activity stabilizes and gradually declines but not into the normal range for several weeks to months [70–72]. In the cat, extrahepatic bile duct obstruction results in a twofold increase within 2 days, as much as a fourfold increase within 1 week, and up to a ninefold increase in serum ALP activity within 2 to 3 weeks [33,41,69,73]. Thereafter, activity stabilizes and gradually declines but usually not into the normal range; the declining enzyme activity coordinates with developing biliary cirrhosis. Cats with experimentally induced incomplete biliary tree occlusion developed ALP values approximately 50% lower than those observed with complete common duct occlusion [41]. In contrast, even partial (experimental) occlusion of the biliary tree in the dog causes marked increases in total serum ALP activity [69–72,74–76]. Inflammatory disorders involving biliary or canalicular structures or disorders compromising bile flow increase serum ALP activity secondary to membrane inflammation or disruption and local bile acid accumulation. In the dog and cat, however, similar magnitudes of serum ALP activities develop in spontaneous intrahepatic cholestasis as compared with disease or obstruction involving the extrahepatic biliary structures; the reader is referred to Figs. 12 and 15. Consequently, ALP activity cannot differentiate between intra- and extrahepatic cholestatic disorders.

Many extrahepatic and primary hepatic conditions enhance production of L-ALP. In the cat, the syndrome of hepatic lipidosis is associated with profound increases in total ALP activity and marked jaundice. A considerable number of disorders leading to inappetence usually precede development of this potentially lethal syndrome [77]. Although the underlying mechanisms provoking high serum ALP activity have not been proven, they likely involve canalicular dysfunction or compression.

In the dog, primary hepatic inflammation as well as systemic infection or inflammation and exposure to steroidogenic hormones may induce a vacuolar hepatopathy [78]. When severe, this disorder also may impose a cholestatic effect on the liver. Although initially well characterized as a glucocorticoid-initiated lesion, it is now well established that nearly 50% of dogs with this syndrome lack overt exposure to glucocorticoids or other steroidogenic substances [78]. Chronically ill dogs may produce the G-ALP isozyme secondary to stress-induced endogenous glucocorticoid release. Chronically ill dogs with this lesion (lacking exogenous glucocorticoid exposure) often demonstrate normal dexamethasone suppression and corticotropin responses. In some dogs, however, this lesion signals the presence of atypical adrenal hyperplasia associated with abnormal sex hormone production (especially 17-OH progesterone). Diagnostically, canine vacuolar hepatopathy is usually first recognized because of markedly increased serum ALP activity in a dog lacking signs of liver disease. This curious physiologic response to endogenous or exogenous steroidogenic hormones is characterized histologically [78–81]. Hepatocytes become markedly distended (up to a 10-fold cell expansion) with glycogen, and in severe cases (rare), cell swelling can impose intrahepatic sinusoidal hypertension and canalicular compression, leading to jaundice and even abdominal effusion. There is no consistent relation between the magnitude of serum ALP activity, the presence of high G-ALP activity, and the histologic lesion. Unfortunately, G-ALP is not useful for syndrome characterization, because this isozyme can become the predominant enzyme in dogs treated with glucocorticoids; dogs with spontaneous or iatrogenic hyperadrenocorticism; dogs with hepatic or nonhepatic neoplasia; and, most importantly, dogs with many different chronic illness, including primary liver disease [43,82,83].

In controlled studies of this syndrome, induction of ALP occurred as early as 1 week after initiation of daily administration of prednisone (2 mg/kg once daily) [83], as early as 2 days after daily administration of prednisone (4.4 mg/kg once daily) [79], and as early as 3 days after daily administration of dexamethasone (2.2 mg/kg once daily) [36]. The initial increase in ALP activity is attributable to the L-ALP isozyme; thereafter, however, the G-ALP becomes the dominant isozyme (Fig. 16) [62,63]. Different magnitudes of enzyme activity develop depending on the type of glucocorticoid administered, the dose given, and the individual patient response [81,82]. Increases in total serum ALP activity attributable primarily to G-ALP usually exceed those associated with liver or bone isoenzymes. In one study, after consecutive daily administration of prednisone at a dose of 4.4 mg/kg and treatment discontinuation, dogs reached a maximum ALP activity of 64-fold normal by day 20 (see Fig. 16) [79]. The ALP activity gradually decreased to 8-fold normal by day 56. This study is relevant to clinical practice, because a commonly prescribed immunosuppressive dose of prednisone was used. In conclusion, the

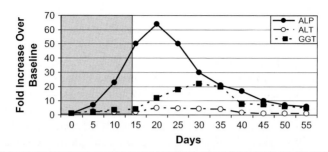

Fig. 16. Response depicting the fold increase from baseline of ALP, ALT, and γ-glutamyltransferase (GGT) activity in dogs given prednisone at a dose of 4.4 mg/kg/d (*gray shaded area*). Enzyme activity continued to increase after treatment was suspended. Data represent mean values. (*Data from* Badylak SF, Van Vleet JF. Sequential morphologic and clinicopathologic alterations in dogs with experimentally induced glucocorticoid hepatopathy. Am J Vet Res 1981;42;1310–18.)

production of G-ALP does not imply that a dog treated with cortisone has iatrogenic hyperadrenocorticism, a suppressed pituitary adrenal axis, or a clinically important vacuolar hepatopathy.

By comparison, the feline liver is relatively insensitive to glucocorticoids. Administration of prednisolone (5 mg twice daily) to normal cats for 30 days failed to elicit an increase in ALP activity in serum or liver tissue [40]. When cats received prednisolone at a dose of 2 mg/kg once daily for 16 days, changes in serum ALP also did not develop or were minor. Morphologic hepatocellular alterations are rare and minor in most studies but were suggested to reflect hepatocellular vacuolar glycogen retention in some cats in two investigations [84,85].

In dogs, serum total ALP activity and L-ALP isozyme also may be induced by administration of certain anticonvulsants (phenobarbital, primidone, and phenytoin) [86,87]. Induced ALP activity usually increases 2- to 6-fold normal activity. During a 30-day study of drug administration to normal dogs, phenytoin (22 mg/kg administered orally three times daily) produced a uniform small increase in serum ALP activity; phenobarbital (4.4 mg/kg administered orally three times daily) produced peak serum enzyme activity 30-fold normal by 24 days, which thereafter declined; and primidone (17.6 mg/kg administered orally three times daily) produced a 5-fold increase in serum ALP activity by day 28. Healthy dogs receiving combination therapy (eg, primidone, phenytoin) developed ALP increases ranging from 2- to 12-fold normal, with some receiving high-dose phenobarbital developing ALP activity 30- to 40-fold greater than the normal range. In contrast to the dog, the administration of phenobarbital (0.25 grain twice daily) for 30 days in cats failed to elicit an increase in serum or liver tissue ALP activity [40].

γ-GLUTAMYLTRANSFERASE

γ-Glutamyltransferase (γ-GT) is a membrane-bound glycoprotein that catalyzes the transpeptidation and hydrolysis of the γ-glutamyl group of glutathione

(GSH) and related compounds. Through this reaction, it plays a critical role in cellular detoxification and confers resistance against several toxins and drugs. Its reactions with GSH are essential for maintaining the balance of the intracellular redox status. Because GSH is the most abundant intracellular nonprotein thiol and is involved in a myriad of biologic processes (eg, regulation of the intracellular redox status, conjugation of electrophile toxins), γ-GT plays a formidable role in intermediary metabolism. In addition to ensuring cysteine availability, γ-GT hydrolyzes GSH-related compounds, including leukotriene-C, prostaglandins, and several γ-glutamyl amino acids, and catalyzes the transfer of the γ-glutamyl group from GSH to dipeptides and amino acids [88]. The latter transamidation process is essential for amino acid transport (recovery) in the renal tubules. Experimental work suggests that expression of γ-GT is regulated by glucocorticoids, and it is known that induction phenomena increase hepatic γ-GT production [89]. Because acute exposure to oxidative stress increases gene transcription for γ-GT synthesis, it seems that the regulation of γ-GT synthesis is an adaptive response protecting cells against oxidative injury. Although enhanced synthesis contributes to the serum γ-GT activity, cholestatic disorders promote the bile acid solubilization and release of γ-GT from its membrane anchor.

A connection between γ-GT and neoplastic transformation has been made repeatedly in the liver as well as in experimental carcinogenesis. It has been proposed that increased γ-GT expression may contribute to tumor progression and formation of aggressive and drug-resistant phenotypes. One theory suggests that increased γ-GT synthesis enhances the capacity for GSH-mediated drug detoxification, thereby limiting drug residence time. An alternative argument is that enhanced γ-GT activity increases availability of cysteinyl-glycine residues that complex extracellularly with drug metabolites, augmenting formation of reactive oxygen species [90].

The highest tissue concentrations of γ-GT in the dog and cat are located in the kidney and pancreas, with lesser amounts in the liver, gallbladder, intestine, spleen, heart, lungs, skeletal muscle, and erythrocytes [71,80,91]. Serum γ-GT activity is largely derived from the liver, although there is considerable species variation in its localization within this organ. Hepatic microsomal localization has been proven for γ-GT in the dog, where it is associated with canaliculi, bile ducts, and zone 1 (periportal) hepatocytes [72,76,91]. Increased serum γ-GT activity reflects enhanced synthesis in the liver and regurgitation of eluted enzyme from membrane surfaces. The diagnostic performance of γ-GT has been scrutinized in clinical patients with and without liver disease [71,92–94].

Experimental study of serum γ-GT activity in dogs and cats undergoing acute severe diffuse necrosis has shown no change or only mild increases (1- to 3-fold normal) that resolve over the ensuing 10 days. In the dog, extrahepatic bile duct obstruction causes serum γ-GT activity to increase from 1- to 4-fold normal within 4 days and from 10- to 50-fold normal within 1 to 2 weeks. Thereafter, values may plateau or continue to increase as high as 100-fold normal [17,71,76]. In the cat with extrahepatic bile duct obstruction, serum γ-GT activity may increase up to 2-fold normal within 3 days, 2- to 6-fold normal within 5 days, 3- to 12-fold normal within a week, and 4- to 16-fold normal within 2 weeks [18,69].

Glucocorticoids and certain other microsomal enzyme inducers may stimulate γ-GT production in the dog similar to their influence on ALP. Administration of dexamethasone (3 mg/kg once daily) or prednisone (4.4 mg/kg intramuscularly once daily) increased γ-GT activity within 1 week to 4- to 7-fold normal and up to 10-fold normal within 2 weeks [75,79,80]. Increased synthesis of γ-GT secondary to glucocorticoid administration is surmised to involve the liver. In comparison to glucocorticoid induction, dogs treated with phenytoin or primidone (anticonvulsants) develop only a modest increase in serum γ-GT activity up to 2- or 3-fold normal, unless they also develop idiopathic anticonvulsant hepatotoxicosis [95].

Some cats with advanced necroinflammatory liver disease, major bile duct obstruction, or inflammatory intrahepatic cholestasis develop a larger fold increase in γ-GT activity relative to ALP (see Fig. 12) [93]. In other species, cholestasis is known to enhance enzyme synthesis as well as membrane release of γ-GT. It remains undetermined whether glucocorticoids or other enzyme inducers clinically influence serum γ-GT in the cat. It is noteworthy that the normal range for feline serum γ-GT activity is much narrower and lower than in the dog. Thus, interpreting feline γ-GT activity using the canine reference range leads to erroneous conclusions. Additionally, because of the comparatively low γ-GT activity in feline serum, assay sensitivity may be a problem if reagent solubility is less than optimum (ie, low γ-GT activity may be undetected).

Remarkably increased γ-GT values have been observed in dogs and cats with primary hepatic or pancreatic neoplasia. Although a unique γ-GT isozyme is associated with HCCA in human beings, it has not been determined that a similar paraneoplastic phenomenon occurs in dogs or cats. In people, γ-GT is also used in surveillance for hepatic metastasis; however, it does not seem to be suitable for this application in the dog or the cat.

The sensitivity of γ-GT for the detection of liver disease is summarized in Fig. 17. Like ALP, γ-GT lacks specificity in differentiating between pavenchymal hepatic disease and occlusive biliary disease. It is not as sensitive in the dog as ALP but does have higher specificity [34,93]. In cats with inflammatory liver disease, γ-GT is more sensitive but less specific than ALP, and these two enzymes perform best when interpreted simultaneously [93]. The prediction that hepatic lipidosis has developed secondary to necroinflammatory liver disease, biliary duct occlusion, or pancreatic disease can be made by examining the relative increase in γ-GT compared with ALP. Necroinflammatory disorders involving biliary structures, the portal triad, or the pancreas are associated with a fold increase in γ-GT exceeding that of ALP in the cat (see Fig. 12). With the exclusion of these underlying disorders, cats with hepatic lipidosis have higher fold increases in ALP relative to γ-GT (this is illustrated by data presented in Figs. 12, 13, and 17). The mechanism for this difference presumably is the involvement of duct epithelium in inflammatory processes (biliary ducts

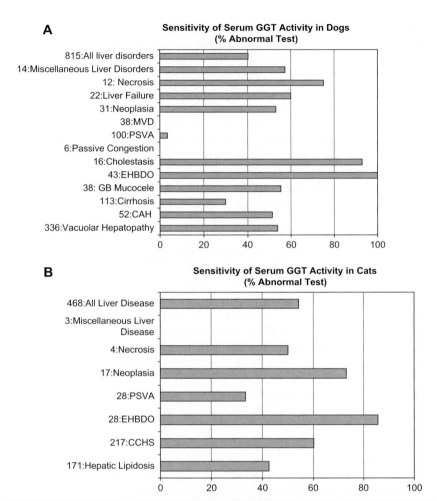

Fig. 17. Sensitivity of serum γ-GT (GGT) activity for the detection of hepatobiliary syndromes in the dog (*A*) and cat (*B*). The number preceding the disease description indicates the number of cases included. Miscellaneous liver disorders included disorders that could not be classified in other categories and for which there were fewer than five cases. CAH, chronic "active" hepatitis; CCHS, cholangitis or cholangiohepatitis syndrome of cats; EHBDO, extrahepatic bile duct occlusion; GB, gallbladder; MVD, microvascular dysplasia; PSVA, portosystemic vascular anomaly. All diagnoses were confirmed by liver biopsy or definitive imaging studies in dogs with a PSVA. (*Data from* the New York State College of Veterinary Medicine, Cornell University, Ithaca, NY, 2006.)

and pancreatic ducts), because these likely have greater potential for γ-GT production.

Neonatal animals of several species, including the dog but not the cat, develop high serum γ-GT activity secondary to colostrum ingestion, as discussed in detail elsewhere in this article [96–98].

LACTATE DEHYDROGENASE

LDH has a wide tissue distribution in all species. The highest tissue concentrations, in descending order, occur in the skeletal muscle, heart, and kidney, with lesser amounts in the intestine, liver, lung, and pancreas [99]. Each tissue has been shown to contain at least five isozymes [99]. LDH_5 predominates in the liver and is believed to be a major contributor to serum LDH activity. Serum biochemistry profiles report total LDH, however, negating the utility of this enzyme for detection of hepatobiliary abnormalities. High LDH activity is often observed in animals with diffuse severe hepatic necrosis or inflammation, myositis or muscle trauma, and lymphosarcoma external to the liver.

ARGINASE

Arginase is considered to be a liver-specific enzyme because it exists in higher concentrations in hepatocytes than in any other tissue (Fig. 18). It functions as a major catalyst of the urea cycle, with large quantities located in mitochondria. With severe hepatic insults, damaged mitochondrial membranes acutely release preformed arginase into the systemic circulation [15,100]. Tissue concentrations of arginase in several species have demonstrated specificity for the liver [15]. Although a simplified method for arginine analysis has adapted the test for clinical practice, its utility is limited to detection of severe acute hepatic insults because of its transient appearance in serum. Consequently, it has never gained the popularity needed to support its routine measurement economically.

With acute severe necrosis, ALT and arginase are immediately released from hepatocytes, causing a marked sharp rise in their serum activities [100,101]. If plasma arginase and transaminase activities become persistently increased, a progressive necrotizing lesion is surmised [15]. In dogs and cats, experimentally induced acute hepatic necrosis with CCl_4^- causes a 500- to

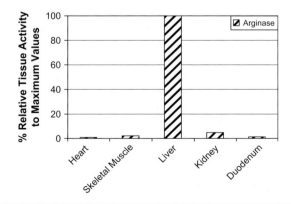

Fig. 18. Comparative tissue distribution of arginase in a dog. (*Data from* Mia AS, Koger HD. Comparative studies on serum arginase and transaminases in hepatic necrosis in various species of domestic animals. Vet Clin Pathol 1979;8:9–15.)

1000-fold increase in arginase that persists for only 2 to 3 days. During recovery, sustained increases in serum transaminase activity reflect continued enzyme leakage and longer plasma $t_{1/2}$. During recovery, leakage of transaminases but not arginase continues, with ALT and AST activity persisting for 1 week or longer [15,101,102].

Dogs treated with dexamethasone (3 mg/kg once daily for 11 days) developed a transient 5- to 8-fold increase in arginase activity by day 4 [74]. With treatment chronicity, a steady increase in serum arginase was maintained. At study termination (day 12), serum arginase activity was 10-fold normal [74]. Glucocorticoid induction of catabolic adaptations may contribute to this high arginase activity, as reported in other species [15,74,100–103].

SORBITOL DEHYDROGENASE
Sorbitol dehydrogenase (SDH) is a cytosolic enzyme released during hepatic degeneration or necrosis or secondary to altered membrane permeability. The concentration of SDH is greater in the liver than in all other tissues [3]. Although it may be a useful test for recognition of hepatocellular injury, it offers no advantage over determination of serum ALT activity. There also is concern over its lability in vitro as compared with ALT. Consequently, there has been little use of this enzyme in small animal diagnostic enzymology.

SERUM ENZYME PATTERNS IN EXTRAHEPATIC BILE DUCT OCCLUSION AND ACUTE HEPATIC NECROSIS
Typical enzyme patterns in dogs and cats sequentially sampled after experimentally induced acute hepatic necrosis (CCl_4^- initiated) and surgically created extrahepatic bile duct obstruction are displayed in Figs. 19 and 20, showing routinely used enzymes as well as arginase and SDH.

ENZYMATIC MARKERS OF HEPATIC NECROSIS: THE HEALING PHASE
Hepatic necrosis, a common reaction to liver injury, is followed by a reactive regenerative response driven by a multitude of interacting cells, cytokines, regulatory factors, and extracellular matrix molecules [104,105]. The extent or degree of hepatic regeneration depends on the type of injurious agent or event, the nature of the underlying liver disease, and the number of affected cells. Hepatocytes and bile duct epithelium maintain the potential to replicate when challenged with appropriate stimuli. A population of pluripotential cells (oval cells) also contributes to parenchymal and ductal repair [104,105]. Cell replication during the healing process explains the delayed onset or late phase and sustained increases in liver enzymes (especially of the membrane-affiliated ALP and γ-GT) after severe diffuse hepatocellular injury.

INFLUENCE OF AGE ON LIVER ENZYME ACTIVITY
Age-appropriate reference intervals for serum liver enzyme activity are essential in puppies and kittens. Plasma enzyme activities of ALP and γ-GT in the

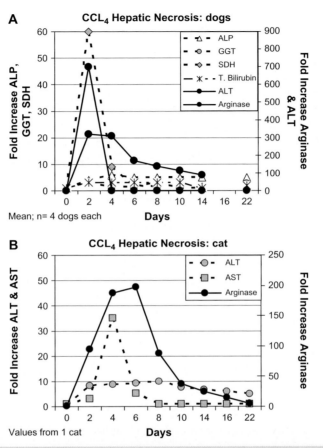

Fig. 19. Enzymology associated with severe acute hepatic necrosis induced by administration of CCl_4^- in dogs and a cat and chronic bile duct obstruction in dogs showing the clinical utility of routinely measured enzymes as well as arginase and SDH. (*Data from* Noonan NE, Meyer DJ. Use of plasma arginase and gamma-glutamyl transpeptidase as specific indicators of hepatocellular or hepatobiliary disease in the dog. Am J Vet Res 1979;40:942–47; and Mia AS, Koger HD. Comparative studies on serum arginase and transaminases in hepatic necrosis in various species of domestic animals. Vet Clin Pathol 1979;8:9–15.)

dog and cat are significantly influenced by age. Neonates have markedly higher serum enzyme activities than adults (Fig. 21) [4,96–98]. These differences reflect physiologic adaptations during the transition from fetal and neonatal life stages, colostrum ingestion, maturation of metabolic pathways, growth effects, differences in volume of distribution and body composition, and nutrition [97]. An important factor influencing serum liver enzyme activity in neonatal dogs and cats is the enteric absorption of colostral macromolecules during the first day of life (Fig. 22) [96–98]. In neonates, serum activity of ALP, AST, CK, and LDH usually increases greatly during the first 24 hours after

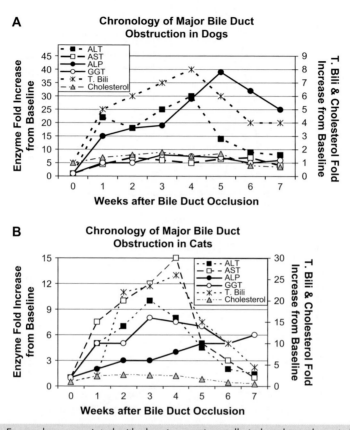

Fig. 20. Enzymology associated with chronic experimentally induced extrahepatic bile duct occlusion in the dog and cat. GGT, γ-glutamyltransferase.

birth. In kittens, serum activity of ALP, CK, and LDH exceeds adult values through 8 weeks of age. Early increases in AST, CK, and LDH are proposed to reflect muscle trauma associated with birth, whereas ALP activity reflects the bone isoenzyme (early bone growth). Serum ALP markedly increases in 1-day-old puppies and kittens subsequent to colostrum ingestion, however [96,97]. One-day-old pups (n = 5) had serum γ-GT activities 29-fold greater and ALP activities 5-fold greater than 2- and 7-month-old dogs [4]. Further study demonstrated increased ALP (30-fold) and γ-GT (100-fold) in 1- to 3-day-old pups relative to normal adult dogs [96]. Significant differences between γ-GT and ALP activities developed between colostrum-deprived and suckling pups within 24 hours. At 10 and 30 days after birth, serum γ-GT and ALP activities were less than values before suckling in all pups. Colostrum had substantially higher γ-GT and ALP activities compared with bitches' serum (γ-GT was 100-fold greater and ALP was 10-fold greater in colostrum and milk than in serum

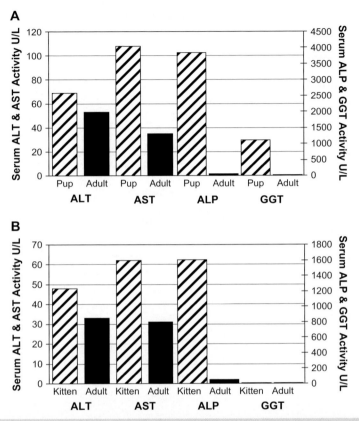

Fig. 21. The serum transaminase, ALP, and γ-GT (GTT) activity in 1- to 3-day-old puppies and kittens compared with healthy adults. (*Data from* references 96–98.)

through day 10). By day 30, γ-GT and ALP activity in milk was less than before suckling had started. Although a marked influence of colostrum on serum ALP activity in neonatal kittens also occurs, the effect on γ-GT is modest (see Fig. 22) [97,98]. The analysis of milk and colostrum (Fig. 23) from bitches and queens demonstrates the remarkable concentrations of enzymes imbibed and resorbed by the 1-day-old neonate.

HEPATOCELLULAR CARCINOMA AND SERUM ENZYME ACTIVITY

Dogs with HCCA or hepatoma commonly display increased serum liver enzyme activity. In those with HCCA, serum ALP or ALT is most often increased. More than one liver enzyme is elevated in 90% of such dogs (Fig. 24); the median magnitude of serum enzyme abnormalities in dogs with massive HCCA is shown in Fig. 25 [106]. In dogs undergoing successful surgical resection, liver enzymes normalize within 2 to 3 weeks. Markedly

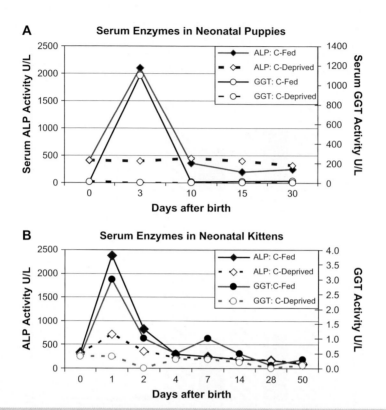

Fig. 22. The serum transaminase, ALP, and γ-GT (GTT) activity in 1- to 3-day-old puppies and kittens compared with healthy adults. The sharp increase in ALP and GTT in dogs and ALP in cats is derived from colostrum. (*Data from* Refs. [96–98].)

increased ALT and AST activity indicates a poor prognosis, because high transaminase activity reflects aggressive tumor behavior, fast growth rate, and large tumor size. High serum bile acid concentrations indicate loss of functional hepatic mass, release of cytokines from neoplastic cells causing paraneoplastic cholestasis, or invasion or compression of the porta hepatis compromising circulation or bile flow. The full spectrum of biochemical abnormalities commonly associated with hepatic dysfunction or liver disease (eg, hypoalbuminemia, hypercholesterolemia, coagulopathy) is infrequently encountered in dogs with massive HCCA. These tumors may be nodular (approximately 29%) or diffuse (approximately 10%) and more commonly involve the left liver lobes. Although large-volume surgical debulking is difficult, a median survival time of 4 years has been reported [106]. Dogs not undergoing surgical tumor excision had a median survival time of 270 days [106]. Prognostic indicators for poor surgical outcome include high ALT and AST activity and right-sided tumor invasion (right-sided involvement is technically more difficult to extirpate).

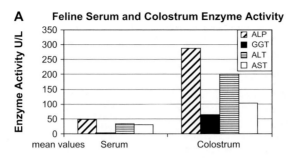

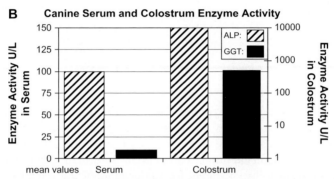

Fig. 23. The relative concentration of transaminases, ALP, and γ-GT (GTT) activity in the serum and colostrum from lactating queens and bitches. (*Data from* Center SA, Randolph JR, Man-Warren T, et al. Effect of colostrums ingestion on gamma-glutamyltransferase and alkaline phosphatase activities in neonatal pups. Am J Vet Res 1991;52:499–504; and Crawford PC, Levy JK, Werner LL. Evaluation of surrogate markers for passive transfer of immunity in kittens. J Am Vet Med Assoc. 2006;228:1038–41.)

SUMMARY

Abnormalities in liver enzymes are commonly encountered in clinical practice. Knowledgeable assessment requires a full understanding of their pathophysiology and provides an important means of detecting the earliest stage of many serious hepatobiliary disorders. The best interpretations are achieved using an integrated approach, combining historical and physical findings with routine and specialized diagnostic procedures and imaging studies. In some cases, liver enzyme abnormalities initiate early assessment of liver function using serum or urine bile acid determinations that help to prioritize the need for liver biopsy and definitive disease characterization. Several unique syndromes have been described in which liver enzymes direct diagnostic and therapeutic decisions. These include the ALP/γ-GT ratio in the feline hepatic lipidosis syndrome, the induction of the glucocorticoid-ALP isoenzyme with steroidogenic hormones, the development of the canine vacuolar hepatopathy syndrome, the apparent paraneoplastic association between ALP and some mammary neoplasia, the prognostic value of transaminases in dogs with massive HCCA, the origin

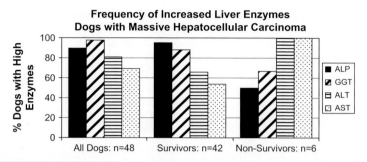

Fig. 24. Frequency of increased serum enzyme activities in dogs with large-volume or "massive" HCCA. GGT, γ-glutamyltransferase. (*Data from* Liptak JM, Dernell WS, Monnet E, et al. Massive hepatocellular carcinoma in dogs: 48 cases (1992-2002). J Am Vet Med Assoc 2004;225:1225–30.)

of increased serum ALP in hyperthyroid cats, the inhibition of transaminase synthesis by certain toxins (eg, aflatoxin, microcystin) blunting evidence of lethal hepatocellular injury, and the influence of colostrum ingestion on serum enzyme activity in neonatal puppies and kittens. Information in this article provides the foundation, by example, for understanding the reliability of single time point enzyme measurements, the value of sequential measurements, the importance of interpreting the activity of enzymes in light of their $t_{1/2}$ and tissue of origin, and the influence of the induction phenomenon. Understanding the contribution of the proliferative reparative process that follows severe liver injury explains why a protracted increase in cholestatic enzyme activity is observed during the recovery process.

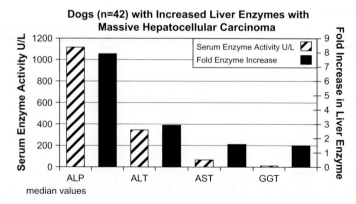

Fig. 25. Magnitude of increased serum enzyme activities in dogs with large-volume or "massive" HCCA. (*Data from* Liptak JM, Dernell WS, Monnet E, et al. Massive hepatocellular carcinoma in dogs: 48 cases (1992-2002). J Am Vet Med Assoc 2004;225:1225-30.)

References

[1] Van Hoof VO, Deng JT, DeBrow ME. How do plasma membranes reach the circulation. Clin Chim Acta 1997;266:23–31.

[2] Nagode LA, Frajola WJ, Loeb WF. Enzyme activities of canine tissues. Am J Vet Res 1966;27:1385–93.

[3] Zinkl JG, Bush RM, Cornelius CE, et al. Comparative studies on plasma and tissue sorbitol, glutamic, lactic, and hydroxybutyric dehydrogenase and transaminase activities in the dog. Res Vet Sci 1971;12:211–4.

[4] Keller P. Enzyme activities in the dog: tissue analyses, plasma values, and intracellular distribution. Am J Vet Res 1981;41:575–82.

[5] Rej R. Aminotransferases in disease. Clin Lab Med 1989;9(4):667–87.

[6] Valentine BA, Blue JT, Shelley SM, et al. Increased serum alanine aminotransferase activity associated with muscle necrosis in the dog. J Vet Intern Med 1990;4:140–3.

[7] Bolter CP, Critz JB. Changes in plasma enzyme activity elicited by running exercise in the dog. Proc Soc Exp Biol Med 1974;145:1359–62.

[8] Loegering DJ, Critz JB. Effect of hypoxia and muscular activity on plasma enzyme levels in dogs. Am J Physiol 1971;220:100–4.

[9] Heffron JJA, Bomzon L, Pattinson RA. Observations on plasma creatine phosphokinase activity in dogs. Vet Rec 1976;98:338–40.

[10] Dossin O, Rives A, Germain C, et al. Pharmacokinetics of liver transaminases in healthy dogs: potential clinical relevance for assessment of liver damage. [abstract 152, ACVIM Annual Meeting], J Vet Intern Med 2005.

[11] Nilkumhang P, Thornton JR. Plasma and tissue enzyme activities in the cat. J Small Anim Pract 1979;20:169–74.

[12] Kamimoto Y, Horiuchi S, Tanase S, et al. Plasma clearance of intravenously injected aspartate aminotransferase isozymes: evidence for preferential uptake by sinusoidal liver cells. Hepatology 1985;5:367–75.

[13] Horiuchi S, Kamimoto Y, Morino Y. Hepatic clearance of rat liver aspartate aminotransferase isozymes: evidence for endocytotic uptake via different binding sites on sinusoidal liver cells. Hepatology 1985;5:376–82.

[14] Cornelius CE, Kaneko JJ. Serum transaminases activities in cats with hepatic necrosis. J Am Vet Med Assoc 1960;137:62–6.

[15] Cornelius CE, Douglas GM, Gronwall RR, et al. Comparative studies on plasma arginase and transaminases in hepatic necrosis. Cornell Vet 1963;53:181–91.

[16] Van Vleet JF, Alberts JO. Evaluation of liver function tests and liver biopsy in experimental carbon tetrachloride intoxication and extrahepatic bile duct obstruction in the dog. Am J Vet Res 1968;29:2119–31.

[17] Noonan NE, Meyer DJ. Use of plasma arginase and gamma-glutamyl transpeptidase as specific indicators of hepatocellular or hepatobiliary disease in the dog. Am J Vet Res 1979;40:942–7.

[18] Spano JS, August JR, Henderson RA, et al. Serum gamma-glutamyltranspeptidase activity in healthy cats and cats with induced hepatic disease. Am J Vet Res 1983;44:2049–53.

[19] Dixon MF, Fulker MJ, Walker BE, et al. Serum transaminases levels after experimental paracetamol-induced hepatic necrosis. Gut 1975;16:800–7.

[20] Strombeck DR, Harrold D, Rogers Q, et al. Plasma amino acids, glucagon, and insulin concentrations in dogs with nitrosamine-induced hepatic disease. Am J Vet Res 1983;44:2028–36.

[21] King JM. The correlation of liver function tests with the hepatic lesion in dogs fed toxic peanut meal [PhD thesis]. College of Veterinary Medicine, Cornell University, 1963.

[22] Solter P, Liu Z, Guzman R. Decreased hepatic ALT synthesis is an outcome of subchronic microcystin-LR toxicity. Toxicol Appl Pharmacol 2000;164:216–20.

[23] Schaeffer MC, Rogers QR, Buffington CA, et al. Long-term biochemical and physiologic effects of surgically placed portacaval shunts in dogs. Am J Vet Res 1986;47:346–55.

[24] St. Omer VV, McKnight ED 3rd. Acetylcysteine for treatment of acetaminophen toxicosis in the cat. J Am Vet Med Assoc 1980;176:911–3.

[25] Savides MC, Oehme FW, Nash SL, et al. The toxicity and biotransformation of single doses of acetaminophen in dogs and cats. Toxicol Appl Pharmacol 1984;74(1):26–34.

[26] Hjelle JJ, Grauer GF. Acetaminophen-induced toxicosis in dogs and cats. J Am Vet Med Assoc 1986;188:742–6.

[27] Ortega L, Landa Garcia JI, Torres Garcia A, et al. Acetaminophen-induced fulminant hepatic failure in dogs. Hepatology 1985;5:673–6.

[28] Panella C, Makowka L, Barone M, et al. Effect of ranitidine on acetaminophen-induced hepatotoxicity in dogs. Dig Dis Sci 1990;35:385–91.

[29] Wigton DH, Kociba GJ, Hoover EA. Infectious canine hepatitis: animal model for viral induced disseminated intravascular coagulation. Blood 1976;47:287–96.

[30] Boyd JW. The mechanisms relating to increases in plasma enzymes and isoenzymes in diseases of animals. Vet Clin Pathol 1983;12:9–24.

[31] Morino Y, Kagamiyama H, Wada J. Immunochemical distinction between glutamic-oxalo-acetic transaminases from soluble and mitochondrial fractions of mammalian tissues. J Biol Chem 1964;239:943–4.

[32] Mia AS, Koger HD. Direct colorimetric determination of serum arginase in various domestic animals. Am J Vet Res 1978;173:1381–3.

[33] Center SA, Baldwin BE, Tennant B, et al. Hematologic and biochemical abnormalities associated with induced extrahepatic bile duct obstruction in the cat. Am J Vet Res 1983;44:1822–9.

[34] Abdelkader SV, Hauge JG. Serum enzyme determination in the study of liver disease in dogs. Acta Vet Scand 1986;27:50–70.

[35] Center SA, ManWarren T, Slater MR, et al. Evaluation of twelve-hour preprandial and two-hour postprandial serum bile acids concentrations for diagnosis of hepatobiliary disease in dogs. J Am Vet Med Assoc 1991;199:217–26.

[36] Dillon AR, Spano JS, Powers RD. Prednisolone induced hematologic, biochemical, and histological changes in the dog. J Am Anim Hosp Assoc 1980;16:831–7.

[37] Solter PF, Hoffmann WE. Canine corticosteroid-induced alkaline phosphatase in serum was solubilized by phospholipase activity in vivo. Am J Physiol 1995;32:G278–86.

[38] Solter PF, Hoffmann WE. Solubilization of liver alkaline phosphatase isoenzyme during cholestasis in dogs. Am J Vet Res 1999;66:1010–5.

[39] Hawrylak K, Stinson RA. The solubilization of tetrameric alkaline phosphatase from human liver and its conversion into various forms by phosphatidylinositol phospholipase C or proteolysis. J Biol Chem 1988;263:14368–73.

[40] Hoffmann WE, Renegar WE, Dorner JL. Alkaline phosphatase and alkaline phosphatase isoenzymes in the cat. Vet Clin Pathol 1977;6:21–4.

[41] Everett RM, Duncan JR, Prasse KW. Alkaline phosphatase, leucine aminopeptidase and alanine aminotransferase activities with obstructive and toxic hepatic disease in cats. Am J Vet Res 1977;38:963–6.

[42] Foster DJ, Thoday KL. Tissue sources of serum alkaline phosphatase in 34 hyperthyroid cats: a qualitative and quantitative study. Res Vet Sci 2000;68:89–94.

[43] Hoffmann WE. Diagnostic value of canine serum alkaline phosphatase and alkaline phosphatase isoenzymes. J Am Anim Hosp Assoc 1977;13:237–41.

[44] Hoffmann WE, Dorner JL. Separation of isoenzymes of canine alkaline phosphatase by cellulose acetate electrophoresis. J Am Anim Hosp Assoc 1975;11:283–5.

[45] Saini PD, Peavy GM, Hauser DE, et al. Diagnostic evaluation of canine serum alkaline phosphatase by immunochemical means and interpretation of results. Am J Vet Res 1978;39:1514–8.

[46] Hoffmann WE, Dorner JL. Disappearance rate of intravenous injected canine alkaline phosphatase isoenzymes. Am J Vet Res 1977;38:1553–5.

[47] Hoffman WE, Dorner JL. Serum half-life of intravenously injected intestinal and hepatic alkaline phosphatase isoenzymes in the cat. Am J Vet Res 1977;38:1637–9.

[48] Bengmark S, Olsson R. Elimination of alkaline phosphatases from serum in dog after intravenous injection of canine phosphatases from bone and intestine. Acta Chir Scand 1974;140:1–6.

[49] Everett RM, Duncan JR, Prasse KW. Alkaline phosphatase in tissues and sera of cats. Am J Vet Res 1977;38:1533–8.

[50] Horney BS, Farmer AJ, Honor DJ, et al. Agarose gel electrophoresis of alkaline phosphatase isoenzymes in the serum of hyperthyroid cats. Vet Clin Pathol 1994;23:98–102.

[51] Peterson ME, Kintzer PP, Cavnagh PG, et al. Feline hyperthyroidism: pretreatment clinical and laboratory evaluation of 131 cases. J Am Vet Med Assoc 1983;183:103–10.

[52] Thoday KL, Mooney CT. Historical, clinical and laboratory features of 126 hyperthyroid cats. Vet Rec 1992;132:257–64.

[53] Mundy GR, Shapiro JL, Bandelin JG, et al. Direct stimulation of bone resorption by thyroid hormones. J Clin Invest 1976;58:529–34.

[54] Cooper DS, Kaplan MM, Ridgway C, et al. Alkaline phosphatase isoenzyme patterns in hyperthyroidism. Ann Intern Med 1979;90:164–8.

[55] Rhone DP, Berlinger FG, White FM. Tissue sources of elevated serum alkaline phosphatase activity in hyperthyroid patients. Am J Clin Pathol 1980;74:381–6.

[56] Tibl L, Patrick AW, Leslie P, et al. Alkaline phosphatase isoenzymes in plasma in hyperthyroidism. Clin Chem 1989;35:1427–30.

[57] Archer FJ, Taylor SM. Alkaline phosphatase bone isoenzyme and osteocalcin in the serum of hyperthyroid cats. Can Vet J 1996;37:735–9.

[58] Barber PJ, Elliott J. Study of calcium homeostasis in feline hyperthyroidism. J Small Anim Pract 1996;37(12):575–82.

[59] Wiedmeyer CE, Solter PE, Hoffmann WE. Kinetics of mRNA expression of alkaline phosphatase isoenzymes in hepatic tissues from glucocorticoid-treated dogs. Am J Vet Res 2002;63:1089–95.

[60] Wiedmeyer CE, Solter PE, Hoffmann WE. Alkaline phosphatase expression in tissues from glucocorticoid-treated dogs. Am J Vet Res 2002;63:1083–8.

[61] De Brow ME, Roels F, Nouwen EJ, et al. Liver plasma membrane: the source of high molecular weight alkaline phosphatase in human serum. Hepatology 1985;5:118–28.

[62] Sanecki RK, Hoffmann WE, Dorner JL, et al. Purification and comparison of corticosteroid-induced and intestinal isoenzymes of alkaline phosphatase in dogs. Am J Vet Res 1990;51:1964–8.

[63] Sanecki RK, Hoffmann WE, Gelberg HB, et al. Subcellular location of corticosteroid-induced alkaline phosphatase in canine hepatocytes. Vet Pathol 1987;24:296–301.

[64] Seetharam S, Sussman NL, Komoda T, et al. The mechanism of elevated alkaline phosphatase activity after bile duct ligation in the rat. Hepatology 1986;6:374–80.

[65] Hadley SP, Hoffman WE, Kuhlenschmidt MS, et al. Effect of glucocorticoids on ALP, ALT, and GGT in cultured dog hepatocytes. Enzyme 1990;43:89–90.

[66] Hatoff DE, Hardison WGM. Bile acid dependent secretion of alkaline phosphatase in rat bile. Hepatology 1982;2:433–9.

[67] Karayannopoulou M, Koutinas AF, Polizopoulou ZS, et al. Total serum alkaline phosphatase activity in dogs with mammary neoplasms: a prospective study on 79 natural cases. J Vet Med A Physiol Pathol Clin Med 2003;50:501–5.

[68] Hamilton JM, Wright J, Kight D. Alkaline phosphatase levels in canine mammary neoplasia. Vet Rec 1973;93:121–3.

[69] Meyer D. Serum gamma-glutamyltransferase as a liver test in cats with toxic and obstructive hepatic disease. J Am Anim Hosp Assoc 1983;19:1023–6.

[70] Shull RM, Hornbuckle W. Diagnostic use of serum gamma-glutamyltransferase in canine liver disease. Am J Vet Res 1979;40:1321–4.

[71] Guelfi JF, Braun JP, Bernard P, et al. Value of so-called cholestasis markers in the dog. Res Vet Sci 1982;33:309–12.

[72] Aronsen KF, Hagerstand F, Norden JG. Enzyme studies in dogs with extra-hepatic biliary obstruction. Scand J Gastroenterol 1968;3:355–68.

[73] McLain DL, Nagode LA, Wilson GP, et al. Alkaline phosphatase and its isoenzymes in normal cats and in cats with biliary obstruction. J Am Anim Hosp Assoc 1978;14:94–9.

[74] DeNovo RC, Prasse KW. Comparison of serum biochemical and hepatic functional alterations in dogs treated with corticosteroids and hepatic duct ligation. Am J Vet Res 1983;44:1703–9.

[75] Stein TA, Rurns GP, Wise L. Diagnostic value of liver function tests in bile duct obstruction. J Surg Res 1989;46:226–9.

[76] Kokot F, Grzybek H, Kuska J. Experimental studies on gamma-glutamyl transpeptidase. IV. Histoenzymatic and biochemical changes in parenchymatous hepatitis in rabbits and in obstructive jaundice in dogs. Acta Med Pol 1975;6:379–88.

[77] Center SA. Feline hepatic lipidosis. Vet Clin North Am Small Anim Pract 2005;35:225–69.

[78] Sepesy LM, Center SA, Randolph JF, et al. Vacuolar hepatopathy in dogs: 336 cases (1993-2005). J Am Vet Med Assoc 2006;229:246–52.

[79] Badylak SF, Van Vleet JF. Sequential morphologic and clinicopathologic alterations in dogs with experimentally induced glucocorticoid hepatopathy. Am J Vet Res 1981;42:1310–8.

[80] Badylak SF, Van Vleet JF. Tissue gamma-glutamyl transpeptidase activity and hepatic ultrastructural alterations in dogs with experimentally induced glucocorticoid hepatopathy. Am J Vet Res 1982;43:649–55.

[81] Dillon AR, Sorjonen DC, Powers RD, et al. Effects of dexamethasone and surgical hypotension on hepatic morphologic features and enzymes of dogs. Am J Vet Res 1983;44:1996–9.

[82] Hoffmann WE, Dorner JL. A comparison of canine normal hepatic alkaline phosphatase and variant alkaline phosphatase of serum and liver. Clin Chim Acta 1975;62:137–42.

[83] Dorner JL, Hoffman WE, Long GB. Corticosteroid induction of an isoenzyme of alkaline phosphatase in the dog. Am J Vet Res 1974;35:1457–8.

[84] Middleton DJ, Watson AD, Howe CJ, et al. Suppression of cortisol responses to exogenous adrenocorticotrophic hormones and the occurrence of side effects attributable to glucocorticoid excess in cats during therapy with megestrol acetate and prednisolone. Can J Vet Res 1986;51:60–5.

[85] Fulton R, Thrall MA, Weiser MG, et al. Steroid hepatopathy in cats. [platform presentation]. Proc Am Soc Vet Clin Pathol 1988;23.

[86] Sturtevant F, Hoffman WE, Dorner JL. The effect of three anticonvulsant drugs and ACTH on canine serum alkaline phosphatase. J Am Anim Hosp Assoc 1977;13:754–7.

[87] Bunch SE, Castleman WL, Hornbuckle WE, et al. Hepatic cirrhosis associated with long-term anticonvulsant drug therapy in dogs. J Am Vet Assoc 1982;181:357–62.

[88] Ikeda Y, Taniguchi N. Gene expression of γ-glutamyltranspeptidase. Methods Enzymol 2005;401:408–25.

[89] Billon MC, Dupre G, Hanoune J. In vivo modulation of rat hepatic γ-glutamyltransferase activity by glucocorticoids. Mol Cell Endocrinol 1980;18:99–108.

[90] Pompella A, De Tata V, Paolicchi A, et al. Expression of γ-glutamyltransferase in cancer cells and its significance in drug resistance. Biochem Pharmacol 2006;71:231–8.

[91] Braun JP, Benard P, Burgat V, et al. Gamma glutamyl transferase in domestic animals. Vet Res Commun 1983;6:77–90.

[92] Krebs C. Gamma-glutamyltransferase activity in the cat [inaugural dissertation]. Ludwig-Maximilans Universitat, Munchen; 1979. p. 122.

[93] Center SA, Baldwin BH, Dillingham S, et al. Diagnostic value of serum γ-glutamyl transferase and alkaline phosphatase in hepatobiliary disease in the cat. J Am Vet Med Assoc 1986;201:507–10.

[94] Center SA, Slater MR, ManWarren T, et al. The diagnostic efficacy of serum alkaline phosphatase and γ-glutamyl transferase in the dog with histologically confirmed hepatobiliary disease. A study of 270 cases (1980-1990). J Am Vet Med Assoc 1992;201:1258–64.

[95] Bunch SE. Effects of anticonvulsant drugs phenytoin and primidone on the canine liver [thesis]. Cornell University, 1983. p. 81.

[96] Center SA, Randolph JR, ManWarren T, et al. Effect of colostrum ingestion on gamma-glutamyltransferase and alkaline phosphatase activities in neonatal pups. Am J Vet Res 1991;52:499–504.

[97] Levy JK, Crawford PC, Werner LL. Effect of age on reference intervals of serum biochemical values in kittens. J Am Vet Med Assoc 2006;228:1033–7.

[98] Crawford PC, Levy JK, Werner LL. Evaluation of surrogate markers for passive transfer of immunity in kittens. J Am Vet Med Assoc 2006;228:1038–41.

[99] Milne EM, Doxey DL. Lactate dehydrogenase and its isoenzymes in the tissues and sera of clinically normal dogs. Res Vet Sci 1987;43:222–4.

[100] Cargill CF, Shields RP. Plasma arginase as a liver function test. J Comp Pathol 1971;81: 447–54.

[101] Cacciatore L, Antoniello S, Valentino B, et al. Arginase activity, arginine and ornithine of plasma in experimental liver damage. Enzyme 1974;17:269–75.

[102] Ugarte G, Pino ME, Peirano P. Serum arginase activity in subjects with hepatocellular damage. J Lab Clin Med 1960;55:522–9.

[103] Mia AS, Koger HD. Comparative studies on serum arginase and transaminases in hepatic necrosis in various species of domestic animals. Vet Clin Pathol 1979;8:9–15.

[104] Bisgaard HC, Thorgeirsson SS. Hepatic regeneration: the role of regeneration in pathogenesis of chronic liver diseases. Clin Lab Med 1996;16:325–39.

[105] Fausto N. Liver regeneration. J Hepatol 2000;22:19–31.

[106] Liptak JM, Dernell WS, Monnet E, et al. Massive hepatocellular carcinoma in dogs: 48 cases (1992-2002). J Am Vet Med Assoc 2004;225:1225–30.

Vet Clin Small Anim 37 (2007) 335–350

VETERINARY CLINICS
SMALL ANIMAL PRACTICE

LSEVIER
AUNDERS

New Challenges for the Diagnosis of Feline Immunodeficiency Virus Infection

P. Cynda Crawford, DVM, PhD*, Julie K. Levy, DVM, PhD

Department of Small Animal Clinical Sciences, College of Veterinary Medicine,
University of Florida, 2015 SW 16th Avenue, Gainesville, FL 32610, USA

Feline immunodeficiency virus (FIV) infection is one of the most common infectious diseases of domestic cats worldwide. The true prevalence of FIV is unknown because testing is voluntary, results are not reported to a central database, and most screening test results are not confirmed by another technology. Seroprevalence studies have generally relied on convenience testing of healthy cats; sick cats; cats at high risk for exposure; and feral cats in veterinary clinics, animal sheltering facilities, and spay-neuter programs. These studies have shown that the seroprevalence of FIV is highly variable and depends on the age, gender, lifestyle, physical condition, and geographic location of the cat and that the seroprevalence ranges from less than 1% in healthy cats in North America to 44% in sick cats in Japan [1–17]. The most recent FIV seroprevalence study used a prospective cross-sectional survey of 18,038 cats of all ages, lifestyles, and health conditions tested during a single season at 345 veterinary clinics and 145 animal shelters in North America [17]. The overall seroprevalence was 2.5%, and the seroprevalence was higher among cats tested at veterinary clinics (3.1%) than among cats tested at animal shelters (1.7%). The seroprevalence was also higher in adults (4.1%), male cats (3.6%), cats that were sick at the time of testing (6.1%), cats with access to the outdoors (4.3%), and feral cats at animal shelters (3.9%).

Similar to other lentiviral infections, FIV infection is considered to be lifelong, with recovery from infection being extremely rare [18,19]. Cats are typically infected with FIV through biting, but mucosal infection through sexual contact [20–24] and vertical transmission from infected queens to kittens in utero, intrapartum, or by ingestion of colostrum and milk [25–28] is possible. Plasma- and cell-associated viremia occurs during the first 2 months of infection when clinical signs may be apparent, followed by a strong antibody response that correlates with a reduction in viremia and progression to a long period of varying duration and few clinical abnormalities [18,19,23,24,29–32]. During

*Corresponding author. E-mail address: crawfordc@mail.vetmed.ufl.edu (P.C. Crawford).

0195-5616/07/$ – see front matter   Published by Elsevier Inc.
doi:10.1016/j.cvsm.2006.11.011   vetsmall.theclinics.com

the chronic phase of FIV infection, the concentration of circulating viral antigens is lower than the threshold of detection [18,19,23,29,30,32,33]. Therefore, current FIV diagnostic tests rely on detection of FIV antibodies in peripheral blood. Because FIV produces a persistent infection from which few, if any, cats recover, antibody-positive cats are considered to be FIV infected.

Accurate diagnosis of FIV infection is important for uninfected and infected cats. Failure to identify infected cats may lead to inadvertent exposure and transmission of FIV to uninfected cats. Identification and segregation of infected cats is considered to be the most effective method for preventing new infections with FIV. Misdiagnosis of FIV infection in uninfected cats may lead to inappropriate changes in lifestyle and euthanasia. The American Association of Feline Practitioners (AAFP) recommends the use of antibody assays to determine the FIV status of all cats, regardless of age or health status [34,35]. These recommendations include testing of cats when they are first acquired as pets, when their infection status is unknown, after exposure to infected cats, when they have a history of unsupervised outdoor activity, when they reside with infected cats, and when they are sick, regardless of previous test results. Many animal shelters test cats for FIV antibodies before making a decision on eligibility for adoption or euthanasia. Testing of young kittens for FIV antibodies is especially problematic because of passive transfer of immunity. Kittens readily absorb FIV antibodies in colostrum from FIV-infected queens [26,27]. The passively acquired maternal antibodies to FIV result in false-positive FIV diagnostic test results in the kittens. Because detection of FIV antibodies in kittens is considered evidence of exposure to an infected cat (the queen) and possible infection, the AAFP recommends isolation of antibody-positive kittens pending further testing up to 6 months of age [34,35]. Most kittens revert to a negative test result status as the maternal antibodies decay during the first 3 months postpartum. Because logistic and financial issues may limit opportunities for segregation before retesting, kittens are frequently euthanatized after a single positive FIV antibody test result or may not be tested at all to avoid the confusion associated with positive test results.

SEROLOGY TESTS FOR DIAGNOSIS OF FELINE IMMUNODEFICIENCY VIRUS

Two FIV antibody test kits licensed by the US Department of Agriculture (USDA) are currently available for veterinarians in the United States and form the cornerstone of FIV diagnosis. Both are ELISA-based formats that use FIV core proteins $p24^{gag}$ and p15 immobilized on a membrane or plastic well to capture antibodies in whole blood, plasma, or serum [36,37]. One is a lateral-flow ELISA (SNAP FIV Antibody/FeLV Antigen Combo Test, IDEXX Laboratories, Westbrook, Maine) that is commonly used as a point-of-care test at veterinary clinics and animal shelters (Fig. 1). The point-of-care test was determined to have a sensitivity (detection of truly infected cats) of 98.2% and a specificity (detection of truly uninfected cats) of 100% for FIV during licensing trials (M. Dietz, IDEXX Laboratories, personal

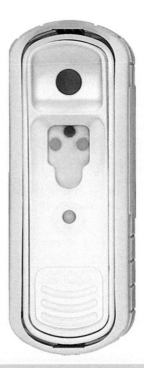

Fig. 1. The lateral-flow ELISA (SNAP FIV Antibody/FeLV Antigen Combo Test; IDEXX Laboratories) for testing cats for FIV antibody and feline leukemia virus (FeLV) antigen. This assay can be used with whole blood, plasma, or serum and is commonly employed as a point-of-care test at veterinary clinics and animal shelters. The window in the center of the device contains the test readout. The center spot is the positive control. This spot turns blue if the assay reagents are active. The blue spot on the left indicates the binding of FIV antibodies in the sample to the immobilized FIV p24^{gag} and p15 antigens in the membrane. The blue spot on the right indicates the binding of FeLV antigen in the sample to immobilized monoclonal antibody to FeLV p27 protein. (*Courtesy of* IDEXX Laboratories, Westbrook, ME; with permission.)

communication, 2005). The other kit is a microwell plate ELISA (PetChek FIV Antibody Test Kit; IDEXX Laboratories) used by reference laboratories for batch testing of large numbers of serum samples (Fig. 2). Studies utilizing older versions of the test kits or tests produced in other countries reported up to 20% false-positive results that were attributable to operator error [38,39] and use of whole-blood samples in the point-of-care test [40]. False-negative results are possible in both assays and occur when cats have not yet seroconverted after recent exposure to FIV or when the concentration of FIV antibodies is less than the detection limit [38,39].

One reference laboratory in the United States (New York State Animal Health Diagnostic Center, Cornell University, Ithaca, New York) offers a kinetic ELISA (KELA) performed in the microwell format. This assay differs from the standard microwell ELISA in that changes in the optical density

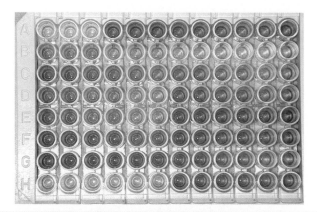

Fig. 2. The microwell ELISA (PetChek FIV Antibody Test Kit; IDEXX Laboratories) for testing cats for antibody to FIV. This assay is used by reference laboratories for batch testing of large numbers of serum samples. The plastic wells contain immobilized FIV p24^{gag} and p15 proteins. Feline serum or plasma is added to the wells, and FIV antibodies, if present, bind to the immobilized antigens. After washing to remove nonspecific proteins, the wells are incubated with a secondary reagent coupled to horseradish peroxidase that binds specifically to FIV antigen-antibody complexes. Addition of the peroxidase substrate results in the development of blue color in the wells that contain FIV antibody. The optical densities in the test wells are compared with the optical densities in the negative and positive control wells to determine seropositivity.

from FIV antigen-antibody reactions are measured repeatedly over time. The laboratory has determined that the FIV KELA provides results equivalent to the specificity and sensitivity of the other serology assays. The advantage over the standard microwell ELISA is the separation of clear negative and positive reactions from equivocal reactions. An equivocal result means that the sample contains some antibody activity but that the optical density is lower than the positive cutoff threshold. Equivocal results are caused by extremely low levels of FIV antibodies or nonspecific reactivity in the cat's serum.

The Western blot test (FIV western blot reagent pack; IDEXX Laboratories) detects antibodies reactive with a range of viral proteins, but it is technically demanding and costly (Fig. 3). Viral proteins from FIV-infected tissue cultures are separated by electrophoresis, transferred to membranes, and incubated with feline serum, followed by incubation with a secondary reagent that detects antibody binding by color development. Serum samples containing antibodies that bind to two or more viral proteins are interpreted as positive for FIV, whereas reactivity with a single viral protein or reactivity with nonviral proteins is considered equivocal or indeterminate [36–39]. The immunofluorescent antibody (IFA) assay (FIV IFA reagent pack; IDEXX Laboratories) is not used as frequently as the Western blot test because interpretation of results is more subjective and operator dependent.

FIV Western Blot

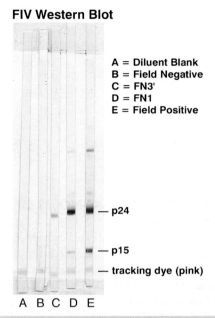

A = Diluent Blank
B = Field Negative
C = FN3'
D = FN1
E = Field Positive

— p24

— p15

— tracking dye (pink)

A B C D E

Fig. 3. The Western blot assay (FIV western blot reagent pack; IDEXX Laboratories) for confirmatory testing of antibody to FIV in feline serum. The negative control is the diluent blank (*A*). The positive controls FN3' (*C*) and FN1 (*D*) are different dilutions of FIV-positive serum. The field negative (*B*) is serum from an uninfected cat. The field positive (*E*) is serum from an FIV-infected cat. Antibodies specific for viral proteins p15 and p24^{gag} are visualized as dark-colored bands. (*Courtesy of* IDEXX Laboratories, Westbrook, ME; with permission.)

In the past, it was reported that ELISA tests were likely to be more sensitive but less specific than Western blot tests for detection of FIV antibodies. As such, ELISA tests were recommended for use as screening tests for diagnosis of FIV infection, but positive results should be confirmed by Western blot analysis or another technology [34,35]. In contrast to older literature, a recent study reported that ELISA tests outperformed other FIV antibody test technologies when plasma collected from 42 FIV-free cats and 41 FIV-infected cats whose FIV status was confirmed by culture was tested. The ELISA was 100% accurate, whereas the Western blot test was 98% sensitive and 98% specific and the IFA was 100% sensitive and 90% specific [33]. Another recent study [41] comparing the accuracy of serology tests for FIV diagnosis also reported that some cats had discordant ELISA, KELA, and Western blot test results and that their true FIV status could not be determined by any combination of serology tests. In addition, 1 uninfected cat had a false-positive result on Western blot analysis. Concurrent infectious diseases have resulted in false-positive or equivocal results in HIV serology tests [42–45], and equivocal FIV serology tests have been documented in cats infected with feline leukemia virus (FeLV), feline infectious peritonitis (FIP), or *Toxoplasma gondii* [39].

In summary, the FIV serology tests are highly accurate, but false or equivocal results can occur from human error, compromised sample integrity, nonspecific reactivity, or low concentrations of antibody in the sample. Positive test results should be confirmed by another type of antibody test. If the results of both tests are positive, there can be high confidence that the cat truly does have FIV antibodies. No single type of FIV antibody test is clearly superior to any other, however, and discordant results require further testing to determine the true FIV status of the cat. Finally, FIV-infected cats may have false-negative test results if blood is collected before seroconversion; thus, the antibody tests should be repeated 2 months later if there is clinical or historical suspicion of virus exposure.

EFFECT OF VACCINATION ON DIAGNOSIS OF FELINE IMMUNODEFICIENCY VIRUS

In 2002, the first FIV vaccine (Fel-O-Vax FIV; Fort Dodge Animal Health, Fort Dodge, Iowa) was licensed. The vaccine is a dual-subtype whole-virus vaccine containing inactivated subtype A (Petaluma) and subtype D (Shizuoka) free virions, virus-infected cells, and an adjuvant [45]. The vaccine is marketed for the prevention of FIV in cats at risk of exposure, such as those that roam outdoors, reside with FIV-infected cats, or have exposure to untested cats. Because the vaccine contains whole virus, cats respond to immunization by producing antibodies that are indistinguishable by current testing methods from those produced during naturally occurring infection [45]. In a recent study to determine the effect of FIV vaccination on the results of serology assays for FIV infection [33], antibodies were detected by the FIV ELISA kits in cats as early as 2 weeks after administration of the first vaccine dose and persisted for at least 1 year. Moreover, the diagnostic performance of the lateral-flow and microwell ELISA kits, the Western blot test, and the IFA was adversely affected by FIV vaccination (Table 1). The sensitivity of all four serology tests

Table 1
Diagnostic performance of four serologic assays for detection of feline immunodeficiency virus (FIV) antibodies in 41 FIV-infected cats, 42 unvaccinated uninfected cats, and 41 FIV vaccinated uninfected cats

		Specificity	
Assay	Sensitivity	Unvaccinated cats	Vaccinated cats
Lateral-flow ELISA	100 (91–100)	100 (92–100)	0 (0–9)[a]
Microwell plate ELISA	100 (91–100)	100 (92–100)	0 (0–9)[a]
Western blot assay	98 (87–100)	98 (87–100)	54 (37–69)[b]
IFA assay	100 (91–100)	90 (77–97)	22 (11–38)[b]

Data are given as mean (95% confidence interval).
   Abbreviation: IFA, immunofluorescent antibody.
   [a,b]In each column, values with different superscripted letters are significantly ($P < .05$) different.
   Data from Levy JK, Crawford PC, Slater MR. Effect of vaccination against feline immunodeficiency virus on results of serologic testing in cats. J Am Vet Med Assoc 2004;225:1560.

was high (98 to 100%) when tested in a defined population of FIV-uninfected, FIV-infected, and FIV-vaccinated cats. Specificity was high in uninfected unvaccinated cats (90%–100%) but was low in uninfected vaccinated cats (0%–54%). Thus, vaccine-induced antibodies cause false-positive results in the FIV serology tests for at least 1 year, but other studies have demonstrated that the antibodies persist for 2 [46] and 3 years (Julie Levy, unpublished observation, 2006).

FIV vaccination also clouds the interpretation of diagnostic testing in kittens. Vaccination of queens against FIV results in passively acquired FIV antibodies in kittens after nursing. Kittens born to FIV-vaccinated queens tested positive for FIV antibodies in the two ELISA kits at 2 days of age [47]. At 8 weeks of age, 55% to 63% of kittens remained antibody-positive, but all kittens were antibody-negative by 12 weeks of age (Fig. 4). Thus, FIV vaccination of queens results in passively acquired FIV antibodies in kittens that frequently persist past the age of weaning when many kittens are tested for FIV before adoption as new pets.

In conclusion, vaccination of cats against FIV with a whole-virus vaccine results in rapid and persistent production of antibodies that are indistinguishable from those used for diagnosis of FIV infection. Therefore, current serologic diagnostic tests for FIV, including the ELISA, KELA, Western blot test, and IFA, cannot distinguish between cats that have antibodies as a result of vaccination against FIV, infection with FIV, or both. The inability of current serologic tests to distinguish between antibodies induced by infection or vaccination has created a diagnostic dilemma for FIV [33,47–49]. Misdiagnosis of infection in vaccinated uninfected cats and kittens born to vaccinated queens

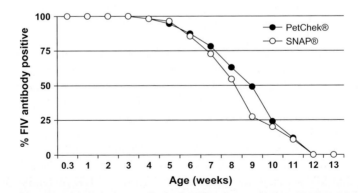

Fig. 4. Percentage of kittens (n = 55) born to FIV-vaccinated queens that tested positive for FIV antibodies in the lateral-flow ELISA (SNAP FIV Antibody/FeLV Antigen Combo Test; IDEXX Laboratories) (*open circles*) and the microwell ELISA (PetChek FIV Antibody Test Kit; IDEXX Laboratories) (*closed circles*) from 2 days through 13 weeks of age. (*Data from* MacDonald K, Levy JK, Tucker SJ, et al. Effects of passive transfer of immunity on results of diagnostic tests for antibodies against feline immunodeficiency virus in kittens born to vaccinated queens. J Am Vet Med Assoc 2004;225:1556.)

may lead to unnecessary changes in lifestyle, ineligibility for adoption, and even euthanasia.

ALTERNATIVE TESTS FOR DIAGNOSIS OF FELINE IMMUNODEFICIENCY VIRUS
Polymerase Chain Reaction

The polymerase chain reaction (PCR) has been promoted as a potential solution for confirming the true FIV status of cats [45,50]. PCR assays can diagnose FIV infection in cats by identifying virus-infected cells in the blood. PCR primers are designed to detect specific DNA sequences in a targeted region of the virus genome. The accuracy of PCR depends on precise matching of the primer sequences to highly conserved sequences in the FIV genome while avoiding analogous sequences in other organisms. PCR exponentially amplifies targeted viral DNA sequences until they are present at detectable concentrations. Because diagnostic PCR can detect as few as 1 to 10 copies of viral DNA in a given sample, it is much more sensitive than many other testing methodologies [51]. The high sensitivity of PCR may lead to false-positive results, however, if minute amounts of DNA contamination occur during collection, storage, or processing of samples [52–54]. Stringent sample handling and contamination precautions as well as quality control measures are necessary to minimize false-positive results in PCR assays [52–54]. Sequencing of PCR products to verify the presence of viral sequences helps to identify false-positive reactions [52–54]. False-negative PCR results occur when there is inadequate sample quality, mismatches between primer and virus sequences, an insufficient amount of virus in the blood sample, and inadequate preparation of basic components for the PCR reaction [52–54].

Like other lentiviruses, FIV has a high intrinsic mutation rate in the envelope (*env*) and capsid (*gag*) genes, which has led to the evolution of several genetically distinct subtypes. Sequence divergence in the *env* and *gag* genes ranges up to 26% within a subtype and between subtypes [11,55–64]. There are five well-characterized subtypes of FIV (A–E) based on genetic divergence in the *env* and *gag* genes [11,55–64]. The most common subtypes found in FIV-infected cats in North America are subtypes A, B, and C [58,60,65] (D. Bienzle, personal communication, 2005). Recently, a unique cluster within subtype B has been described in cats from Texas [66]. Subtypes A, B, and C are also found in cats in Europe, Japan, and Australia [55,56,62,64,67–71], whereas subtype C is found in cats in Taiwan and Vietnam [62,72,73]. Subtype D has been identified in FIV-infected cats in Japan and Vietnam [11,57,59,62,69], and subtype E occurs in cats in Argentina [69,74]. Cats may be infected with one subtype only or coinfected with different subtypes [65,75–77] (D. Bienzle, personal communication, 2005). The coexistence of more than one subtype in a particular location raises the possibility of genetic recombination between coinfecting subtypes, creating intersubtype recombinants with novel features that might interfere with diagnostic tests [77]. Recently, A/B and A/C intersubtype recombinants were identified in FIV-infected cats in Canada [65] (D. Bienzle, personal communication, 2005). Additional subtypes and intersubtype recombinants may emerge as more strains of FIV are fully characterized.

Because genetic diversity is high, identification of circulating FIV subtypes and intersubtype recombinants is essential for the development of strategies for diagnosis of FIV infection by PCR. Primers for FIV PCR are often selected based on *env* and *gag* genetic sequences of a few well-characterized FIV strains. How well these *env* and *gag* primers detect the wide variety of genetically divergent FIV strains present in nature is unknown, but false-negative results ranging from 10% to 100% have been reported [51,55,58,78,79]. Little is known about the performance of the FIV PCR tests currently marketed to veterinary practitioners in North America as an alternative to antibody testing for diagnosis of FIV infection. Additionally, none of these available tests have undergone licensing by the USDA.

Recent studies have investigated the diagnostic accuracy of FIV PCR assays offered to veterinarians by research and commercial laboratories in North America. In one study [41], blood samples from a small population of uninfected and FIV-infected cats were submitted to a research laboratory and two reference laboratories in Canada for FIV PCR testing. FIV subtypes A, B, and C were represented in the population of infected cats. The research laboratory used a conventional nested PCR assay with "universal" primers designed from highly conserved sequences in the *gag* gene of FIV subtypes A, B, and C. In addition, all PCR products were sequenced to verify the presence of FIV and to identify false-positive reactions. The technical details of the PCR assays used by the reference laboratories were not described. The research PCR assay correctly identified all uninfected and FIV-infected cats in this study. Both reference laboratory PCR assays misidentified uninfected and infected cats. The two reference laboratory PCR assays correctly identified only 50% and 80% of the infected cats and 70% and 90% of the uninfected cats. Surprisingly, blood samples from healthy dogs were reported as FIV-positive by both reference laboratories.

In another study [80], blood samples from a large defined population of uninfected, FIV-infected, and FIV-vaccinated cats were submitted to three commercial laboratories in the United States and Canada that offer FIV PCR testing to veterinarians for diagnosis of FIV. The FIV-infected cats were infected with subtypes A, B, or C. One laboratory used a real-time PCR assay with primers designed from conserved sequences in the *gag* gene of FIV subtypes A, B, and C. The second laboratory used a conventional nested PCR assay with primer sequences for the *env* and *gag* gene, whereas the third laboratory used a conventional PCR assay that was not nested with primers for the *gag* gene only. None of the laboratories sequenced the PCR products to verify the presence of FIV and detect false-positive reactions. The sensitivity of the PCR assays ranged from 51% to 93% (ie, depending on the laboratory, 7%–49% of infected cats were not detected; Table 2). The specificity ranged from 81% to 100% in unvaccinated cats and from 44% to 95% in FIV-vaccinated cats. False-positive results from all three laboratories were more

Table 2
Sensitivity and specificity (95% confidence intervals) for three commercial polymerase chain reaction assays (PCR1, PCR2, and PCR3) for detection of feline immunodeficiency virus (FIV) infection in FIV-infected cats, unvaccinated uninfected cats, and FIV-vaccinated uninfected cats

	Cats (n)	PCR1	PCR2	PCR3
Sensitivity for FIV-infected cats	41	76[a] (60, 88)	93[b] (80, 98)	51[c] (35, 67)
Specificity for unvaccinated cats	42	100[a] (92, 100)	81[b] (67, 91)	81[b] (66, 91)
Specificity for vaccinated cats	41	95[a] (83, 99)	66[b] (49, 80)	44[c] (26, 58)

[a,b,c]Within a row, values with different superscripted letters are significantly different ($P < .05$).
    Data from Crawford PC, Slater MR, Levy JK. Accuracy of polymerase chain reactions for diagnosis of feline immunodeficiency virus infection in cats. J Am Vet Med Assoc 2005;226:1505.

numerous in FIV-vaccinated cats than in unvaccinated cats. Thus, all three PCR assays misidentified uninfected and infected cats. The laboratory that used the real-time PCR assay had the highest specificity for all uninfected cats (95%) and the lowest false-positive results for vaccinated cats (5%), but the sensitivity was only 76%. The Canadian research laboratory [41] recently tested their conventional nested PCR assay on a mixed population of uninfected, FIV-infected, and FIV-vaccinated cats. Although the assay missed some infected cats, it correctly identified all uninfected cats (D. Bienzle, personal communication, 2006). The high specificity depended on sequencing of PCR products to eliminate false-positive results, however. This underscores the importance of sequence analysis of PCR products for increasing the accuracy of PCR assays.

In conclusion, FIV PCR assays currently marketed to veterinary practitioners by commercial laboratories in North America vary significantly in diagnostic accuracy and do not resolve the diagnostic dilemma resulting from FIV vaccination. The marked genetic diversity makes FIV a challenging target for detection by PCR. High sequence variation, coupled with low numbers of virus-infected cells in the blood during the lengthy asymptomatic phase of infection when most cats are tested, makes reliable PCR detection of FIV infection difficult. In addition, there are marked differences in the numbers of virus-infected cells in the blood between different field isolates [32].

Virus Culture
Recovery of virus from peripheral blood mononuclear cell (PBMC) cultures is considered the "gold standard" for confirmation of FIV infection in cats in research laboratories. Virus culture performed on mixed populations of uninfected, FIV-infected, and FIV-vaccinated cats successfully verified the true status of all cats [33,80]. Although accurate in FIV diagnosis, the virus culture assay was technically demanding and expensive because it relied on isolation of PBMCs from whole-blood samples, removal of CD8+ T cells from the

PBMCs, and culture of the remaining PBMCs with feline CD4+ T cells for amplification of virus replication. The CD8+ T cells were removed because several studies have shown that their antiviral activity inhibits virus replication in culture, at least for well-characterized laboratory strains of FIV [81–83]. In addition to the technical demands and expense, virus culture required 2 weeks for turnaround of results. Thus, although virus culture has been the only reliable and accurate test for differentiation of uninfected, FIV-infected, and FIV-vaccinated cats to date, this assay is not commercially available and the slow turnaround time for results is not practical or timely for cats in animal shelters or for sick cats.

SUMMARY

Vaccination of cats against FIV with a whole-virus vaccine results in rapid and persistent production of antibodies that are indistinguishable from those used for diagnosis of FIV infection. The inability of current serologic tests to distinguish between antibodies induced by infection, vaccination, or both has created a diagnostic dilemma for FIV. FIV PCR assays currently marketed to veterinary practitioners by commercial laboratories in North America vary significantly in diagnostic accuracy and do not resolve the diagnostic dilemma. Virus culture reliably differentiates FIV-infected from uninfected cats but is too technical, expensive, and slow for reference laboratories to use as the first-line diagnostic test for FIV.

The AAFP guidelines recommend testing of all cats for FIV, including sick cats, kittens and adults before adoption, and cats whose lifestyle puts them at risk for virus exposure. In addition, many animal sheltering facilities use the ELISA FIV antibody tests to screen cats for FIV before making a decision on eligibility for adoption or euthanasia. Diagnosis of FIV can literally be a life or death sentence for millions of cats; thus, diagnostic accuracy is of utmost importance.

All cats should still be screened with the ELISA kits because of their high specificity. Because the prevalence of FIV is low in cats in North America [17] and vaccination against FIV is a relatively uncommon practice, most cats test negative, indicating that they are neither infected nor vaccinated. Cats with potential exposure to FIV-infected cats that initially test negative should be retested in 2 months because of the time required for seroconversion after infection, however. The real dilemma is what confirmatory test to use for cats that are positive for FIV antibodies in the initial testing. Commercial FIV PCR assays may produce false-positive and false-negative results. One ideal strategy for improved confirmatory testing of seropositive cats would be performance of an FIV PCR test with PCR product sequencing to rule out false-positive reactions. To the authors' knowledge, there is no reference or commercial laboratory in North America that offers this testing approach. Another strategy would be performance of an FIV PCR assay on cultures of blood samples instead of directly on blood samples. Culture may quickly amplify the virus to a quantity detectable by PCR. This approach successfully identified cats experimentally infected with puma lentivirus when the virus content in the blood was too low for direct detection by PCR [84]. Sequencing of products obtained by PCR analysis of virus cultures would still be optimal to rule out false-positive results. There are no reference or commercial laboratories that offer this strategy, however.

In conclusion, there are no diagnostic tests available for veterinary practitioners at the present time to resolve the diagnostic dilemma posed by use of whole-virus vaccines for protection of cats against FIV. There is a great need for development of commercially available rapid diagnostic tests that conform to differentiation of infected from vaccinated animals (DIVA) standards.

References

[1] Yamamoto JK, Hansen H, Ho EW, et al. Epidemiologic and clinical aspects of feline immunodeficiency virus infection of cats from the continental United States and Canada and possible mode of transmission. J Am Vet Med Assoc 1989;194:213–20.

[2] Fisch H, Altman NH. Feline immunodeficiency virus infection in a population of pet cats from southeastern Florida. J Vet Diagn Invest 1989;1:339–42.

[3] Shelton GH, Waltier RM, Connor SC, et al. Prevalence of feline immunodeficiency virus and feline leukemia virus infections in pet cats. J Am Anim Hosp Assoc 1989;25:7–12.

[4] Grindem CB, Corbett WT, Ammerman BE. Seroepidemiologic survey of feline immunodeficiency virus infection in cats of Wake County, North Carolina. J Am Vet Med Assoc 1989; 194:226–8.

[5] Ishida T, Washizu T, Toriyabe K, et al. Feline immunodeficiency virus infection in cats of Japan. J Am Vet Med Assoc 1989;194:221–5.

[6] O'Connor TP, Tonelli QJ, Scarlett JM. Report of the National FeLV/FIV Awareness Project. J Am Vet Med Assoc 1991;199:1348–53.

[7] Bandecchi P, Matteucci D, Baldinotti F, et al. Prevalence of feline immunodeficiency virus and other retroviral infections in sick cats in Italy. Vet Immunol Immunopathol 1992;31: 337–45.

[8] Hitt ME, Spangler L, McCarville C. Prevalence of feline immunodeficiency virus in submissions of feline serum to a diagnostic laboratory in Atlantic Canada. Can Vet J 1992;33: 723–6.

[9] Courchamp F, Pontier D. Feline immunodeficiency virus: an epidemiological review. C R Acad Sci Paris 1994;317:1123–34.

[10] Malik R, Kendall K, Cridland J, et al. Prevalences of feline leukaemia virus and feline immunodeficiency virus infections in cats in Sydney. Aust Vet J 1997;75:323–7.

[11] Hohdatsu T, Motokawa K, Usami M, et al. Genetic subtyping and epidemiological study of feline immunodeficiency virus by nested polymerase chain reaction restriction fragment length polymorphism analysis of the gag gene. J Virol Methods 1998;70:107–11.

[12] Lee IT, Levy JK, Gorman SP, et al. Prevalence of feline leukemia virus infection and serum antibodies against feline immunodeficiency virus in unowned free-roaming cats. J Am Vet Med Assoc 2002;220:620–2.

[13] Gibson KL, Keizer K, Golding C. A trap, neuter, and release program for feral cats on Prince Edward Island. Can Vet J 2002;43:695–8.

[14] Luria BJ, Levy JK, Lappin MR, et al. Prevalence of infectious diseases in feral cats in northern Florida. J Feline Med Surg 2004;6:287–96.

[15] Moore GE, Ward MP, Dhariwal J, et al. Use of a primary care veterinary medical database for surveillance of syndromes and diseases in dogs and cats [abstract]. J Vet Intern Med 2004;18:386.

[16] Little SE. Feline immunodeficiency virus testing in stray, feral, and client-owned cats in Ottawa. Can Vet J 2005;46:898–901.

[17] Levy JK, Scott HM, Lachtara JL, et al. Seroprevalence of feline leukemia virus and feline immunodeficiency virus infection among cats in North America and risk factors for seropositivity. J Am Vet Med Assoc 2006;228:371–6.
[18] Yamamoto JK, Sparger E, Ho EW, et al. Pathogenesis of experimentally induced feline immunodeficiency virus infection in cats. Am J Vet Res 1988;49:1246–58.
[19] Pedersen NC, Yamamoto JK, Ishida T, et al. Feline immunodeficiency virus infection. Vet Immunol Immunopathol 1989;21:111–29.
[20] Jordan HL, Howard JG, Bucci JG, et al. Horizontal transmission of feline immunodeficiency virus with semen from seropositive cats. J Reprod Immunol 1998;41:341–57.
[21] Jordan HL, Liang Y, Hudson LC, et al. Feline immunodeficiency virus is shed in semen from experimentally and naturally infected cats. AIDS Res Hum Retroviruses 1998;10:1087–92.
[22] Stokes CR, Finerty S, Gruffydd-Jones TJ, et al. Mucosal infection and vaccination against feline immunodeficiency virus. J Biotechnol 1999;20:213–21.
[23] Burkhard MJ, Mathiason CK, Bowdre T, et al. Feline immunodeficiency virus Gag- and Env-specific immune responses after vaginal versus intravenous infection. AIDS Res Hum Retroviruses 2001;17:1767–78.
[24] Burkhard MJ, Mathiason CK, O'Halloran K, et al. Kinetics of early FIV infection in cats exposed via the vaginal versus intravenous route. AIDS Res Hum Retroviruses 2002;18: 217–26.
[25] O'Neil LL, Burkhard MJ, Hoover EA. Frequent perinatal transmission of feline immunodeficiency virus by chronically infected cats. J Virol 1996;70:2894–901.
[26] Sellon RK, Jordan HL, Kennedy-Stoskopf S, et al. Feline immunodeficiency virus can be experimentally transmitted via milk during acute maternal infection. J Virol 1994;68:3380–5.
[27] Allison RW, Hoover EA. Feline immunodeficiency virus is concentrated in milk early in lactation. AIDS Res Hum Retroviruses 2003;19:245–53.
[28] Allison RW, Hoover EA. Covert vertical transmission of feline immunodeficiency virus. AIDS Res Hum Retroviruses 2003;15:421–34.
[29] English RV, Nelson P, Johnson CM, et al. Development of clinical disease in cats experimentally infected with feline immunodeficiency virus. J Infect Dis 1994;170:543–52.
[30] Diehl LJ, Mathiason-DuBard CK, O'Neil LL, et al. Longitudinal assessment of feline immunodeficiency virus kinetics in plasma by use of a quantitative competitive reverse transcriptase PCR. J Virol 1995;69:2328–32.
[31] Hokanson RM, TerWee J, Choi IS, et al. Dose response studies of acute feline immunodeficiency virus PPR strain infection in cats. Vet Microbiol 2000;76:311–27.
[32] Pedersen NC, Leutenegger CM, Woo J, et al. Virulence differences between two field isolates of feline immunodeficiency virus (FIV-APetaluma and FIV-CPGammar) in young adult specific pathogen free cats. Vet Immunol Immunopathol 2001;79:53–67.
[33] Levy JK, Crawford PC, Slater MR. Effect of vaccination against feline immunodeficiency virus on results of serologic testing in cats. J Am Vet Med Assoc 2004;225:1558–61.
[34] Levy J, Richards J, Edwards D, et al. Feline retrovirus testing and management. Compendium on Continuing Education for the Practicing Veterinarian 2001;23:652–7.
[35] Levy J, Richards J, Edwards D, et al. 2001 Report of the American Association of Feline Practitioners and Academy of Feline Medicine Advisory Panel on feline retrovirus testing and management. J Feline Med Surg 2003;5:3–10.
[36] O'Connor TP, Tanguay S, Steinman R, et al. Development and evaluation of immunoassay for detection of antibodies to the feline T-lymphotropic lentivirus (feline immunodeficiency virus). J Clin Microbiol 1989;27:474–9.
[37] Tonelli QJ. Enzyme-linked immunosorbent assay methods for detection of feline leukemia virus and feline immunodeficiency virus. J Am Vet Med Assoc 1991;199:1336–9.
[38] Barr MC, Pough MB, Jacobson RH, et al. Comparison and interpretation of diagnostic tests for feline immunodeficiency virus infection. J Am Vet Med Assoc 1991;199:1377–81.
[39] Barr MC. FIV, FeLV, and FIPV: interpretation and misinterpretation of serological test results. Semin Vet Med Surg (Small Anim) 1996;11:144–53.

[40] Hartmann K, Werner RM, Egberink H, et al. Comparison of six in-house tests for the rapid diagnosis of feline immunodeficiency and feline leukaemia virus infections. Vet Rec 2001; 149:317–20.

[41] Bienzle D, Reggeti F, Wen X, et al. The variability of serological and molecular diagnosis of feline immunodeficiency virus infection. Can Vet J 2004;45:753–75.

[42] Hsia J. False-positive ELISA for human immunodeficiency virus after influenza vaccination. J Infect Dis 1993;167:989–90.

[43] Challakere K, Rapaport MH. False-positive human immunodeficiency virus type I ELISA results in low-risk subjects. West J Med 1993;159:214–5.

[44] Wai CT, Tambyah PA. False-positive HIV-1 ELISA in patients with hepatitis B. Am J Med 2002;112:737.

[45] Uhl EW, Heaton-Jones TG, Pu R, et al. FIV vaccine development and its importance to veterinary and human medicine: a review. FIV vaccine 2002 update and review. Vet Immunol Immunopathol 2002;90:113–32.

[46] Berlinski PJ, Gibson JK, Forester NJ, et al. Further investigation into the increased susceptibility of cats to feline immunodeficiency virus (FIV) after vaccination with parenteral vaccines [abstract]. J Vet Intern Med 2003;17:382.

[47] MacDonald K, Levy JK, Tucker SJ, et al. Confounding of FIV diagnostic testing in kittens by passive transfer of immunity from vaccinated queens. J Am Vet Med Assoc 2004;225: 1554–7.

[48] Richards JR. Feline immunodeficiency virus vaccine: implications for diagnostic testing and disease management. Biologicals 2005;33:215–7.

[49] Little S. Feline immunodeficiency virus: complications of testing and vaccination. Advances in Small Animal Medicine and Surg 2006;19:1–3.

[50] Connell S. Manufacturer addresses concerns about FIV vaccine. J Am Vet Med Assoc 2003;222:149.

[51] Leutenegger CM, Klein D, Hoffmann-Lehmann R, et al. Rapid feline immunodeficiency virus provirus quantitation by polymerase chain reaction using the TaqMan fluorogenic real-time detection system. J Virol Methods 1999;78:105–16.

[52] Hartley JL, Rashtchian A. Dealing with contamination: enzymatic control of carryover contamination in PCR. PCR Methods Appl 1993;3:10–4.

[53] Bastien P, Chabbert E, Lachaud L. Contamination management of broad-range or specific PCR: is there any difference? J Clin Microbiol 2003;41:2272.

[54] Borst A, Box AT, Fluit AC. False-positive results and contamination in nucleic acid amplification assays: suggestions for a prevent and destroy strategy. Eur J Clin Microbiol Infect Dis 2004;23:289–99.

[55] Steinrigl A, Klein D. Phylogenetic analysis of feline immunodeficiency virus in Central Europe: a prerequisite for vaccination and molecular diagnostics. J Gen Virol 2003;84: 1301–7.

[56] Rigby MA, Holmes EC, Pistello M, et al. Evolution of structural proteins of feline immunodeficiency virus: molecular epidemiology and evidence of selection for change. J Gen Virol 1993;74:425–36.

[57] Maki N, Miyazawa T, Fukasawa M, et al. Molecular characterization and heterogeneity of feline immunodeficiency virus isolates. Arch Virol 1992;123:29–45.

[58] Bachmann MH, Mathiason-Rubard C, Learn GH, et al. Genetic diversity of feline immunodeficiency virus: dual infection, recombination, and distinct evolutionary rates among envelope sequence clades. J Virol 1997;71:4241–53.

[59] Nishimura Y, Goto Y, Pang H, et al. Genetic heterogeneity of env gene of feline immunodeficiency virus obtained from multiple districts in Japan. Virus Res 1998;57: 101–12.

[60] Sodora DL, Shaer EG, Kitchell BE, et al. Identification of three feline immunodeficiency virus (FIV) env gene subtypes and comparison of the FIV and human immunodeficiency virus type 1 evolutionary patterns. J Virol 1994;68:2230–8.

[61] Inoshima Y, Miyazawa T, Kohmoto M, et al. Cross virus neutralizing antibodies against feline immunodeficiency virus genotypes A, B, C, D and E. Arch Virol 1998;143:157–62.

[62] Kakinuma S, Motokawa K, Hohdatsu T, et al. Nucleotide sequence of feline immunodeficiency virus: classification of Japanese isolates into two subtypes which are distinct from non-Japanese subtypes. J Virol 1995;69:3639–46.

[63] Carpenter MA, Brown EW, MacDonald DW, et al. Phylogeographic patterns of feline immunodeficiency virus genetic diversity in the domestic cat. Virology 1998;251:234–43.

[64] Greene WK, Meers J, del Fierro G, et al. Extensive sequence variation of feline immunodeficiency virus env genes in isolates from naturally infected cats. Arch Virol 1993;133: 51–62.

[65] Reggeti F, Bienzle D. Feline immunodeficiency virus subtypes A, B, and C and intersubtype recombinants in Ontario, Canada. J Gen Virol 2004;85:1843–52.

[66] Weaver EA, Collisson EW, Slater M, et al. Phylogenetic analyses of Texas isolates indicate an evolving subtype of the Clade B feline immunodeficiency virus. J Virol 2004;78: 2158–63.

[67] Pistello M, Cammarota G, Nicoletti E, et al. Analysis of the genetic diversity and phylogenetic relationship of Italian isolates of feline immunodeficiency virus indicates a high prevalence and heterogeneity of subtype B. J Gen Virol 1997;78:2247–57.

[68] Greene WK, Meers J, Chadwick B, et al. Nucleotide sequences of Australian isolates of the feline immunodeficiency virus: comparison with other feline lentiviruses. Arch Virol 1993; 132:369–79.

[69] Yamada H, Miyazawa T, Tomonaga K, et al. Phylogenetic analysis of the long terminal repeat of feline immunodeficiency viruses from Japan, Argentina and Australia. Arch Virol 1995;140:41–52.

[70] Duarte A, Marques MI, Tavares L, et al. Phylogenetic analysis of five Portuguese strains of FIV. Arch Virol 2002;147:1061–70.

[71] Duarte A, Tavares L. Phylogenetic analysis of Portuguese feline immunodeficiency virus sequences reveals high genetic diversity. Vet Microbiol 2006;114:25–33.

[72] Inada G, Miyazawa T, Inoshima Y, et al. Phylogenetic analysis of feline immunodeficiency virus isolated from cats in Taiwan. Arch Virol 1997;142:1459–67.

[73] Nakamura K, Suzuki Y, Ikeo K, et al. Phylogenetic analysis of Vietnamese isolates of feline immunodeficiency virus: genetic diversity of subtype C. Arch Virol 2003;148:783–91.

[74] Pecoraro MR, Tomonaga K, Miyazawa T, et al. Genetic diversity of Argentine isolates of feline immunodeficiency virus. J Gen Virol 1996;77:2031–5.

[75] Okada S, Pu R, Young E, et al. Superinfection of cats with feline immunodeficiency virus subtypes A and B. AIDS Res Hum Retroviruses 1994;10:1739–46.

[76] Pistello M, Matteucci D, Cammarota G, et al. Kinetics of replication of a partially attenuated virus and of the challenge virus during a three-year intersubtype feline immunodeficiency virus superinfection experiment in cats. J Virol 1999;73:1518–27.

[77] Kyaw-Tanner MT, Greene WK, Park HS, et al. The induction of in vivo superinfection and recombination using feline immunodeficiency virus as the model. Arch Virol 1994;138: 261–71.

[78] Hohdatsu T, Yamada M, Okada M, et al. Detection of feline immunodeficiency proviral DNA in peripheral blood lymphocytes by the polymerase chain reaction. Vet Microbiol 1992;30:113–23.

[79] Klein D, Janda P, Steinborn R, et al. Proviral load determination of different feline immunodeficiency virus isolates using real-time polymerase chain reaction: influence of mismatches on quantification. Electrophoresis 1999;20:291–9.

[80] Crawford PC, Slater MR, Levy JK. Accuracy of polymerase chain reactions for diagnosis of feline immunodeficiency virus infection in cats. J Am Vet Med Assoc 2005;226:1503–7.

[81] Crawford PC, Papadi GP, Levy JK, et al. Tissue dynamics of CD8 lymphocytes that suppress virus replication in cats infected neonatally with feline immunodeficiency virus. J Infect Dis 2001;184:671–81.

[82] Bucci JG, English RV, Jordan HL, et al. Mucosally transmitted feline immunodeficiency virus induces a CD8$^+$ antiviral response that correlates with reduction of cell-associated virus. J Infect Dis 1998;177:18–25.

[83] Hohdatsu T, Sasagawa T, Yamazaki A, et al. CD8$^+$ T cells from feline immunodeficiency virus (FIV) infected cats suppress exogenous FIV replication of their peripheral blood mononuclear cells in vitro. Arch Virol 2002;147:1517–29.

[84] Sondgeroth K, Leutenegger C, Vande Woude S. Development and validation of puma (*Felis concolor*) cytokine and lentivirus real-time PCR detection systems. Vet Immunol Immunopathol 2005;104:205–13.

Vet Clin Small Anim 37 (2007) 351–372

VETERINARY CLINICS
SMALL ANIMAL PRACTICE

Maximizing the Diagnostic Value of Cytology in Small Animal Practice

Leslie C. Sharkey, DVM, PhD[a],*, Sharon M. Dial, DVM, PhD[b], Michael E. Matz, DVM, MS[c]

[a]Department of Veterinary Population Medicine, College of Veterinary Medicine, University of Minnesota, 1365 Gortner Avenue, St. Paul, MN 55108, USA
[b]Department of Veterinary Science and Microbiology, Arizona Veterinary Diagnostic Laboratory, University of Arizona, 2831 North Freeway, Tucson, AZ 85705, USA
[c]Veterinary Specialty Clinic of Tucson, 4909 North La Canada Drive, Tucson, AZ 85704, USA

Cytologic or histologic evaluation of lesions is a critical component of the diagnostic plan for many patients. Although histologic examination of tissues is considered the "gold standard," cytologic evaluation has several important advantages over biopsy in clinical situations, including relative noninvasiveness, avoidance of anesthesia in unstable patients, lower rates of complications, rapid results, and lower cost. These advantages must be balanced with the potential disadvantages of cytology, which include inconclusive results attributable to low cellularity or artifact and misinterpretation attributable to the absence of tissue architecture. Ideally, clinicians should weigh the choice of biopsy or cytology in the context of the diagnostic performance of cytology versus biopsy for individual tissues and lesions. Likewise, clinicians should be aware of how to maximize their chances of obtaining an accurate cytologic diagnosis. In this article, the authors review the veterinary medical literature to provide perspective on the diagnostic performance of cytology by tissue and lesion type. Based on the results of this review and their own experience as diagnostic pathologists and clinicians, the authors outline obstacles to the optimal use of cytology as a diagnostic tool in small animal practice and how they may be overcome.

This review focuses on articles published within the last 10 years that compare cytologic and histologic diagnoses in dogs and cats, with a breakdown by organ system or tissue. Overall, there is great variation between studies, which complicates comparisons. When reviewing articles that evaluate the diagnostic performance of cytology, the following should be considered:

1. Collection methodology seems to influence results. Some authors exclude from analysis all cytology samples deemed nondiagnostic, whereas others

*Corresponding author. E-mail address: shark009@umn.edu (L.C. Sharkey).

0195-5616/07/$ – see front matter
doi:10.1016/j.cvsm.2006.11.004

include all samples from a given site when analyzing correlations between cytology and histopathology.

2. Criteria used to determine the adequacy of the sample preparation are sometimes not described and cannot be evaluated.

3. Criteria for diagnostic "correlation" may reflect anything from similarity in the basic pathologic process to specific diagnoses, demonstrating looseness in the use of such terms as *diagnostic accuracy, diagnostic performance,* and *correlation.*

4. Some studies attempt to control for interobserver variation in interpretation by having a single pathologist review all samples, whereas others seem to use previously written reports prepared by several different pathologists.

5. Gold standard histologic diagnoses with which cytology results are compared are not perfect. Sample collection method and interobserver variation in interpretation associated with the absence of standardized criteria for evaluation can result in discrepancies in the histologic diagnosis that could have an impact on the correlation with the cytologic diagnosis [1–3].

As the authors review the articles in each area, they comment on the features that may influence interpretation of the results.

SURVEY STUDIES

Several studies have examined the correlation between cytologic and histologic diagnoses by tissue. Cohen and colleagues [4] retrospectively examined the records of 269 cases in which cytologic diagnosis was followed by histopathology. Of these cases, 260 comprised dogs and cats. Details of the methods of collection of cytology and histopathology samples were not available; reports from several clinical and anatomic pathologists were reviewed and compared. Complete agreement was defined as exactly or almost exactly the same diagnosis, and partial agreement was defined as a partially correct diagnosis; for example, "a histopathologic diagnosis of hemangiopericytoma and a cytologic diagnosis of spindle cell tumor." Specimens were considered inadequate if the reports indicated insufficiency, and the cytologic and histopathologic correlations were calculated with and without inclusion of inadequate specimens. Grouping samples from all tissues, complete and partial agreement between cytologic and histopathologic diagnoses was 56.1%, including insufficient cytologic samples, but increased to 63.2%, excluding insufficient samples. By location, combined complete and partial agreement between cytologic and histologic diagnoses was 70.5% for cutaneous lesions, 69.2% for bone lesions, and 33.3% for liver lesions, excluding insufficient samples. False-negative cytology results were more common than false-positive results. The diagnostic accuracy of cytology in this study was somewhat less than that reported in a previous study by Eich and colleagues [5], in which 100 masses from various organ systems were evaluated, 95 of which were collected from dogs and cats. Cytology samples for this prospective study were collected during surgery, with aspirates and impression smears prepared from the same sample submitted for histopathology. A single pathologist in the study by Eich and colleagues [5] classified the cytology results as correct specific diagnosis, correct pathologic process, deferred diagnosis, or incorrect compared with histology. Of the 100 cytology samples, 42% had a correct specific diagnosis, 41% had a correctly identified pathologic process, 1% were inconclusive, and 16% were incorrect compared with histology. Overall "accuracy," defined by combining correct specific diagnosis and correct pathologic process, was 83% versus 63% for the study by Cohen and colleagues [4]. Like the study by Cohen and colleagues [4], Eich and colleagues [5] found that accuracy determined by combining correct specific diagnosis and correct pathologic process varied by tissue, being 91% for skin or subcutaneous lesions, 100% for musculoskeletal lesions, and 67% for gastrointestinal tract lesions. Notably, splenic lesions had the lowest accuracy in the study by Eich and colleagues [5] at 38%. This study's data show consistently higher rates of correlation between cytologic and histologic diagnoses for all tissues compared with the data in the study by Cohen and colleagues [4], which may be attributed to intraoperative collection of cytology samples in the study by Eich and colleagues [5]. This methodology may improve lesion visualization and sample quality and ensures that the cytology and histology samples are collected from the same site. Although no specific methodology was provided in the study by Cohen and colleagues [4], the authors imply that presurgical collection and inconsistent ability to isolate or visualize the lesion may have contributed to lower rates of correlation between cytology and histology results.

CUTANEOUS AND SUBCUTANEOUS LESIONS

Ghisleni and colleagues [6] retrospectively examined the correlation between cytologic and histologic diagnoses for 292 nonmammary cutaneous and subcutaneous masses from dogs and cats. Cytologic samples were prepared from 21- to 22-gauge needle aspiration and were of "adequate quality" for diagnosis in 83.2% of cases as determined by one of two clinical pathologists. Inadequate samples were excluded from analysis. Cytology agreed with biopsy as to the presence or absence of neoplasia in 91% of cases, with all tumors correctly classified as epithelial, mesenchymal, round, or melanoma. There was only one false-positive diagnosis of neoplasia; however, there were 21 false-negative findings. These findings corroborate the findings of Eich and colleagues [5] and Cohen and colleagues [4] that cytologic and histopathologic diagnoses have high rates of concurrence for cutaneous and subcutaneous lesions. The observation that cytology has high specificity and somewhat lower sensitivity for the diagnosis of neoplasia was also noted by Eich and colleagues [5], who found 89% sensitivity and 100% specificity for the cytologic detection of neoplasia for all tissues combined.

LYMPH NODES

Recent large studies evaluating the correlation between cytologic and histologic diagnosis of lymphoma were not found. In general, cytologic diagnosis of lymphoma in cats is thought to be more challenging than in dogs because of less accessible tissue distribution and higher frequency of mature cell types [7].

A prospective comparison of techniques for the detection of metastatic neoplasia in the regional lymph nodes of 44 dogs and cats suspected of having malignant solid tumors showed excellent sensitivity and specificity for aspiration cytology (100% and 96%, respectively) and moderate sensitivity and excellent specificity for needle-core biopsy (64% and 96%, respectively) compared with histologic examination of the excised lymph node [8]. In this study, samples classified as nondiagnostic were excluded from analysis if they contained only blood or stromal cells. Tumor types included 16 carcinomas, 18 sarcomas, and 10 round cell malignancies. Single clinical and anatomic pathologists examined tissue. The superior sensitivity of cytology over needle-core biopsy may have been accounted for by the submission of four cytology smears for each lymph node, whereas only a single needle-core biopsy was submitted per node. The authors note that excisional biopsy revealed metastatic disease in only 36% of animals with palpably enlarged lymph nodes, whereas 20% of patients with normal-sized lymph nodes had metastases. These results are qualitatively similar to those of a retrospective study of lymph node metastases in 12 dogs with oral malignant melanoma, in which 40% dogs had cytologic or histologic evidence of metastases despite the absence of regional lymphadenopathy; many dogs with regional lymphadenopathy had no evidence of metastases [9]. Direct comparison of cytology and histopathology was only possible in six cases; in five (83%) cases, diagnoses were in agreement, and in one (17%) case, the cytology was a false-negative result. Thus, the data suggest that cytologic evaluation of regional lymphoid tissue in patients with cancer is a good way to stage malignancies and should be performed even if lymph nodes are palpably normal.

UROGENITAL

A recent retrospective analysis of 25 adult dogs with prostatic disorders compared cytologic and histopathologic diagnoses [10]. Cytologic samples were obtained by a variety of methods, including ultrasound-guided fine-needle aspiration, intraoperative aspiration, prostatic massage, biopsy imprint, and urine sedimentation, whereas histopathology samples were collected by needle, incisional, or excisional biopsy or at necropsy. Smears were reviewed by the two authors of the article. Grouping all data, including two nondiagnostic cytology preparations, there was 80% concordance between cytology and histology for the diagnosis of inflammation, benign prostatic hyperplasia (BPH), and neoplasia. Discrepant results included two inadequate cytologic specimens, one failure of cytology to detect mild BPH, one failure of cytology to detect paraprostatic transitional cell carcinoma (TCC; likely sampling bias), and one cytologic diagnosis of possible TCC in which biopsy failed to reveal TCC but the presence of TCC was later confirmed at necropsy. The discrepant results were thought to be related to the pathologic process; for example, difficulty in obtaining samples from fibrotic lesions and discerning dysplastic from neoplastic epithelial tissue. This small study did not demonstrate an increased correlation between cytology and histology when cytology samples were collected using ultrasound guidance, but the authors acknowledge that the small number of animals in the study may not have allowed detection of an effect.

RESPIRATORY

A small prospective study of 19 dogs and cats with focal peripheral lung consolidation or mass lesions examined the concordance of ultrasound-guided aspiration cytology and histologic evaluation of surgical biopsy, percutaneous ultrasound-guided biopsy, or postmortem samples [11]. Eleven of these animals had neoplastic lesions, of which 91% were correctly identified as to the presence of neoplasia and the tumor type. One (9%) cytology sample was nondiagnostic. The other 8 dogs and cats had infectious disease; 88% of these patients were diagnosed with inflammation, and in 75%, the infectious agent was correctly identified as blastomycosis or bacteria. One animal (12%) had a nondiagnostic aspirate. Another slightly larger retrospective study of pulmonary parenchymal lesions in 28 dogs and cats compared cytology results collected by ultrasound-guided or blind aspiration, endotracheal wash, pleural fluid, and bronchoalveolar lavage, with biopsy samples collected by means of open thoracotomy, keyhole or transcutaneous ultrasound-guided needle biopsy, or postmortem [12]. Cytologic samples were classified as neoplastic, inflammatory, or nondiagnostic after review by a single pathologist. The sensitivity and specificity of cytology for the detection of neoplasia in this study were 77% and 100%, respectively, and cytopathologic categorization of the neoplasm as carcinoma, sarcoma, histiocytic, or round cell concurred with biopsy results in 79% of patients with neoplasia. The higher numbers of false-negative diagnoses of neoplasia versus false-positive results found in this study mirror the findings of the survey studies. Sixty-seven percent of patients with inflammatory disease had an accurate diagnosis of inflammation by cytology, although 33% of patients with a cytologic diagnosis of inflammatory disease also had neoplastic cells detected in biopsy samples. The overall agreement between cytologic and histologic diagnoses was lower for specimens collected blindly (67%) versus those collected with ultrasound guidance (86%), suggesting that sampling bias may contribute to discrepant results. Nasal brush cytology seems to perform well in the diagnosis of chronic intranasal disease in cats [13]. Agreement between cytologic and histologic (collected by pinch endoscopic or excisional biopsy) diagnosis of neoplasia or inflammation was 87% once insufficiently cellular samples were excluded. There was one false-positive diagnosis of lymphoma in a cat with lymphocytic-plasmacytic rhinitis and six (17%) failures to detect neoplasia, including four benign tumors misclassified as inflammatory or hyperplastic lesions, one adenocarcinoma in which small numbers of suggestive cells were missed, and one small cell lymphoma that was diagnosed as mixed lymphocytic and neutrophilic inflammation. The authors suggested that poorly cellular samples increased the likelihood of a false-negative result for neoplasia.

GASTROINTESTINAL

A prospective study of 218 endoscopically collected paired brush and touch cytology samples and mucosal biopsy samples collected from the stomach, small intestine, and colon of 108 dogs and cats showed that the sensitivity and specificity of cytology compared with mucosal biopsy for the detection of mucosal disease were greater than 80% for all tissues [14,15]. Agreement was defined as the presence or absence of disease, and the authors did not correlate specific diagnoses or severity of lesions between cytologic and histologic samples. Slides were reviewed by two clinical pathologists using a detailed objective cytologic grading system for evaluation of gastrointestinal mucosal cytology samples, which may diminish interobserver variation in interpretation of gastrointestinal cytology. The authors attribute false-negative cytology results (6.9%) to an inability to distinguish mild lymphocytic inflammation from aspiration of normal gut-associated lymphoid tissue, the presence of fibrotic or deeply infiltrative lesions, or the presence of extremely focal lesions that were not sampled during collection. False-positive results (3.2%) were attributed to misinterpretation of mature lymphocyte populations and technical complications.

Cytologic examination of the pancreas is requested with increasing frequency at the University of Minnesota Veterinary Clinical Pathology Laboratory; however, little information is available regarding the performance of cytology to distinguish normal, inflammatory, and neoplastic processes in dogs and cats. One study indicates that cytopathology was helpful in establishing a diagnosis of carcinoma in 10 (83%) of 12 cases of exocrine pancreatic carcinoma in dogs and cats [16].

LIVER

Several recent articles have examined the correlation between cytologic and histologic diagnoses from liver samples. A recent retrospective study by Wang and colleagues [17] includes 97 canine and feline liver samples in which cytology samples were collected by ultrasound-guided fine-needle aspiration and biopsy samples were collected percutaneously (at surgery or necropsy), during laparoscopy, or by unspecified methods. Investigators categorized cytologic and histopathologic diagnoses into normal or primary disease categories, including inflammation, vacuolar hepatopathy, neoplasia, primary cholestasis, portosystemic shunt, cirrhosis, other, and nondiagnostic based on previously written reports. Cytologic diagnoses were in agreement with histopathologic findings in 30% of the canine samples and 51% of the feline samples. The higher agreement for feline samples was attributed to the high prevalence of vacuolar hepatopathy in cats that was readily diagnosed cytologically. Inflammatory disease was correctly identified cytologically in 5 (25%) of 20 canine cases and 3 (27%) of 11 feline cases. A previous study by Roth [18] demonstrated similar difficulty with the cytologic diagnosis of inflammatory disease in the liver, with 55% of the discordant cases being attributed to the presence of inflammatory lesions in histopathologic specimens that were not evident cytologically.

Roth's retrospective study [18] of 56 dogs and cats included only diagnostic cytology samples with paired predominantly core biopsy samples, which the author reviewed blindly and categorized as identical diagnoses (61%), partial agreement (19.5%), and disagreement (19.5%). Information regarding visualization of lesions during the collection of cytology samples was not available. In contrast, a study by Weiss and colleagues [19] suggested better correlation between cytologic and histopathologic diagnoses of inflammation; however, dogs in that study had higher rates of suppurative versus nonsuppurative inflammation compared with the other studies, and re-examination of the data shows that several cases of neoplasia were missed and classified as primarily inflammatory disease. For neoplastic processes, only 22% of the neoplasms diagnosed histologically were detected by cytology in the study by Wang and colleagues [17], suggesting low sensitivity for cytology; however, there were only 2% false-positive results, suggesting good specificity. All three of these studies were retrospective analyses of livers in which cytology and biopsy procedures were performed, and Wang and colleagues [17] astutely observe that cytologic examination of the liver for neoplasia may be better than is indicated by these reports, because cases with a definitive cytologic diagnosis of malignancy may not have had a biopsy performed, introducing negative bias to the studies.

Another factor complicating the interpretation of these studies is the heterogeneous methods used to collect histopathologic specimens. Diagnoses based on histopathologic examination of needle biopsy samples of liver tissue only concur with diagnoses based on examination of larger wedge biopsy samples 48% of the time according to one study of 124 dogs and cats [20]; these differences could introduce variability into the correlation between cytology and biopsy diagnoses of liver lesions. Using a novel approach, Stockhaus and colleagues [21] recently prepared cytologic and histologic samples from needle-core biopsies collected from healthy dogs and dogs with liver disease. Using the histologic diagnoses and cytologic observations, these investigators used statistical regression analysis to construct criteria for the cytologic diagnosis of various liver lesions represented in their population of dogs. The presence of a good control population of normal dogs and the correction for normal and age-related changes were strengths of this study [21,22].

CENTRAL NERVOUS SYSTEM

The cytologic features of canine and feline tumors of the central nervous system have been described based on cytologic preparations from biopsy samples with known histologic diagnoses [23–27]. In one study of brain tumors in 10 euthanized dogs, needle aspirate cytology samples were prepared from brains that had been removed from the cranium. Cytology correctly identified the process as neoplastic in all cases; however, the specific type of tumor only agreed with histology 50% of the time [25]. This study suggests that cytology is a good screening test for neoplasia but that biopsy is required for definitive diagnosis. Another study of intracranial lesions from which cytology and histology samples were collected postmortem from 11 dogs and cats evaluated the impact of smear and staining techniques on the correlation of cytologic and histopathologic diagnoses [24]. For all methods of preparation and all lesions, the overall correlation as to pathologic process or specific diagnosis was 81%. The authors found that modified Wright's stain is preferred and that smear or crush preparations were more diagnostic than touch preparations.

BONE

There is little information in the literature regarding the diagnostic accuracy of bone cytology. An article describing a protocol for CT-guided biopsy procedures indicated that four (80%) of five cytologic diagnoses were confirmed histologically, but details of the correlation were not provided [28]. Another study of ultrasound-guided biopsies of suspected neoplastic lesions of bone described five nondiagnostic cytology samples with a histologic diagnosis of neoplasia and another five in which a cytologic diagnosis of neoplasia was confirmed histologically [29]. A larger study compared the cytologic characteristics of imprint smears collected during surgery from 25 dogs with osteosarcoma with smears from 20 dogs hospitalized for removal of bone implants after uncomplicated fracture healing [30]. Because the diagnosis was already established, the goal was to describe cytologic features that might help to confirm a diagnosis of osteosarcoma. The authors conclude that samples from patients with osteosarcoma contained osteoblasts with clumped chromatin, had more criteria of malignancy, and more frequently had mitoses of osteoblasts.

FLUID ANALYSIS

Use of cytology for the detection of neoplasia in pleural and peritoneal effusions in dogs and cats has been reported to have good sensitivity (64% for dogs and 61% for cats) and excellent specificity (99% for dogs and 100% for cats) in a prospective study based on 183 canine and 156 feline samples [31]. In this study, all diagnoses were confirmed by clinical follow-up or necropsy and all cases of malignancy were confirmed by histopathologic examination. Discrepancies were largely attributed to masking of neoplasia by substantial inflammation or the presence of marked reactive mesothelial hyperplasia, which may be difficult to distinguish from neoplasia. The authors note that tumor cells are difficult to identify in samples in which the packed cell volume (PCV) was greater than 20% and that caution should be exercised with these samples.

Cytology is commonly used to document the presence of septic inflammation in cases of peritonitis. In most cases (90% of cats), bacteria can be detected cytologically; however, in only 10% was the presence of suppurative inflammation with degenerate neutrophils noted to suggest the presence of an infectious etiology in cases of septic peritonitis [32].

Examination of 32 direct smears of synovial fluid from canine joints that were normal (19%) or diagnosed with degenerative joint disease (28%) or inflammatory disease (53%) was used to assess the usefulness of microscopic examination of smears in the classification of joint disease [33]. The study found that examination of direct smears was an inaccurate method of estimating cell counts in synovial fluid, typically resulting in high estimates compared with automated quantitation. Inaccuracy may have been related to clumping of cells in viscous samples; however, significant interobserver variation was described. A strength of this study is that interobserver variation was recorded; however, it should be noted that participants in the study were not pathologists. The article concludes that patient progress should not be monitored by smear estimates of cell count, that smear evaluation had some value in identifying joints with inflammatory disease, but that it is generally not possible to distinguish infectious from immune-mediated joint disease or between normal joints and joints with osteoarthritis.

SUMMARY

Inability to obtain a representative sample is an important source of error in the diagnostic accuracy of cytology and biopsy, and the impact may vary by tissue.

Collection of a representative sample may be facilitated by visualization of lesions during collection, although tissues with a normal gross appearance may contain microscopic lesions. Sample collection issues may influence histopathology and cytology. An excellent recent review of techniques for cytologic sample collection and preparation to increase diagnostic yield is available [34].

Nondiagnostic samples and artifact lower the diagnostic accuracy of cytology and needle biopsy specimens.

Pathologists should clearly communicate the quality of the sample and its impact on the diagnostic accuracy of the results to the clinician.

Cytology has high specificity for the diagnosis of neoplasia; however, concurrent inflammation or low-cellularity samples can lead to errors of interpretation on the part of the pathologist.

Good communication between the clinician and pathologist regarding the nature of the lesion and the clinical and treatment history may help the pathologist to know when to recommend additional diagnostic procedures, such as a repeat aspirate or surgical biopsy.

Read articles describing the diagnostic value of cytology carefully and for detail.

Methods matter. Variation in collection technique has an impact on sample quality, and therefore diagnostic value. Incomplete information describing sample collection methods can be a problem when interpreting studies. Criteria for a diagnostic correlation may reflect anything from a correlation in the basic pathologic process to specific diagnoses. Furthermore, some authors exclude all nondiagnostic cytology samples, whereas other authors include all samples submitted from a given site with resultant discrepant correlations reported for different sampling sites and lesion categories. Retrospective studies may be influenced by bias in the populations of patients that have cytologic and histologic examination of lesions.

Large prospective studies in which cytologic and histologic diagnoses are available for a variety of lesions would enable clinicians to make better choices regarding the diagnostic plans for their patients. These studies should include clear descriptions of methodology to facilitate comparison of results.

MAXIMIZING THE DIAGNOSTIC ACCURACY OF CYTOLOGY

Fine-needle aspiration cytology of mass lesions in most tissues and body cavity fluids can be a sensitive and specific diagnostic procedure. The successful use of cytology depends on four factors: the nature of the lesion, the quality of the specimen, the degree of communication between the veterinarian and the cytologist, and appropriate conflict resolution when cytology and histopathology results are discordant. As previously discussed, cytologic examination of adequately cellular aspirates of cutaneous and subcutaneous lesions has high rates of concurrence with histologic diagnoses. Conversely, the accuracy of aspirate cytology of internal lesions is more affected by the site and method of collection. Aspirates of the liver and spleen have a significantly decreased sensitivity and specificity, which is likely attributable not only to the anatomy of these organs but to the multifocal disease processes often found within them. An understanding of the limitations of cytology and the characteristics of the lesions evaluated leads to realistic expectations for the outcome of the procedure and minimizes frustration. An open line of communication between the clinician and pathologist is an essential part of the diagnostic process. Providing a good clinical history and description of the lesion to the pathologist is required for a thorough interpretation of the cytologic findings just as a good patient history is required for the clinician to interpret the physical examination and other clinical findings fully. The remainder of this article focuses on how to optimize the use of cytology for diagnosis of disease processes.

LESION CHARACTERISTICS

Careful choice of lesions for evaluation increases the chances of obtaining a diagnostic sample. Cytology of the canine mammary gland is a good example of the limitations of cytology in some tissues. In one prospective study, 50% of the mammary lesions had discordant cytologic and histologic diagnoses [35]. Firm lesions that yield minimal material and vascular lesions that yield only peripheral blood require excisional or incisional biopsy. Large solid lesions often have necrotic centers or are heterogeneous. Aspiration of the periphery of the lesion, thus avoiding the central necrosis, or multiple aspirations from separate areas to provide a survey of the possible processes increases the chance of obtaining a diagnostic sample. Multifocal lesions may represent one or multiple processes. Aspiration of one of several lesions does not suffice for a diagnosis of all. It is not uncommon to receive multiple aspirates of subcutaneous masses thought to be lipomas and to find one or two of the lesions to be mast cell tumors or soft tissue sarcomas. Inflamed lesions are a significant challenge because of the secondary responses of involved tissues. Hyperplasia of epithelial and mesenchymal cells can be difficult to differentiate from neoplasia based on cytology. The prudent pathologist is wary of overinterpreting scattered individual cells with characteristics suggestive of neoplasia when there is a significant inflammatory component present. Squamous epithelial cells, fibroblasts, mesothelial cells, and transitional cells can have significant anisocytosis, prominent nucleoli, mitotic figures, and variable nuclear to cytoplasmic ratios, characteristics that overlap with neoplasia. Histologic evaluation of these lesions is usually necessary to confirm the cytologic suspicion of neoplasia.

Well-differentiated neoplastic processes can be difficult to differentiate from normal tissue or benign processes. Because normal lymphoid tissue consists primarily of small lymphocytes, it is usually not possible to make a cytologic diagnosis of small cell lymphoma on a lymph node or splenic aspirate. Differentiating small cell lymphoma from lymphocytic inflammation in a liver aspirate is equally difficult. Although of less practical clinical significance, many of the adnexal tumors can have large keratin-filled cysts that yield large amounts of keratin debris with few viable epithelial cells. Differentiation of a simple epithelial cyst from a benign adnexal tumor can be difficult if the characteristic "ghost cells" indicating matrical keratinization in the trichoepithelioma are not present within the keratin debris. More importantly, differentiating malignant from benign adnexal neoplasia can be difficult on the basis of cytology alone. In many cases, the histologic differentiation of basal cell epithelioma from basal cell carcinoma is based on evidence of invasion into adjacent tissue, scirrhous response, and vascular invasion. These are structural details not evident on cytology.

Ultrasound-guided fine-needle aspirates to assist in limiting sampling bias are recommended for internal lesions or lesions within the deep musculature. It is not within the scope of this article to discuss the fine points of using ultrasound instruments in aspiration cytology. Nevertheless, it is worth mentioning that an inexperienced ultrasonographer may forget that there are three dimensions to consider when performing ultrasound-guided aspirates. Confirmation with a perpendicular plane is recommended to define the lesion dimensions better.

SPECIMEN QUALITY

The quality of a cytologic preparation is based on the number of intact nucleated cells in single or multiple monolayer clusters in the preparation. Preparing good diagnostic samples requires experience and patience. It may be necessary to prepare a dozen smears to obtain a single high-quality diagnostic slide. A light touch when making "squash" or "pull" preparations prevents lysis of fragile neoplastic cells during slide preparation. Highly cellular samples that are too thick to allow evaluation of individual cell nuclear and cytoplasmic characteristics can be as nondiagnostic as samples with low cellularity. "Spatter" preparations, in which the material from the needle is sprayed onto the slide without being spread out, are often too thick and may cause damage to the cellular elements.

Vascular tissues, such as the liver and spleen, are inherently bloody. Submission of a concurrent peripheral blood film or complete blood cell count (CBC) along with the cytology may allow better assessment of inflammation and atypical cells in a hemodiluted sample. Bone marrow evaluation requires submission of the results from a concurrent (same day) CBC. Screening cytologic preparations before submission may be helpful to prevent submission of non-diagnostic samples. It is important to discuss submission of prestained slides with the pathologist to whom the preparations are being sent. Individual pathologists may or may not wish to receive prestained slides. If slides are stained and evaluated in-house, it is recommended that all slides be submitted to the laboratory, including the prestained slides.

The utility of a fluid sample can be compromised greatly by inappropriate handling. Complete fluid analysis consists of a nucleated cell count, total protein determination, and microscopic evaluation. All fluid samples for which a complete fluid analysis is required should be submitted in ethylenediaminetetraacetic acid (EDTA). If a culture is anticipated, a separate sample without EDTA is recommended, because EDTA may inhibit the growth of some microorganisms [36]. Occasionally, fluid sediment preparations of low to moderately cellular samples are submitted in addition to or rather than the native fluid. These samples can be useful when fluid analysis is delayed by transportation. In most cases, nucleate cell counts and total protein determinations do not change significantly within 12 to 24 hours if handled properly. This is not true for cellular morphology. Degenerative changes in the nucleated cells within a sample with delayed evaluation can hinder the interpretation of the cytologic findings; therefore, the sediment preparations submitted with the fluid are often the most useful for morphology. Interpretation of these preparations when the native fluid is not included in the submission requires an additional direct preparation to assist in estimating the cellularity of the native fluid or a nucleated cell count and total solids determination to be provided by the clinician.

COMMUNICATION

The successful interaction between clinicians and pathologists is based on open communication and trust. Previously, an analogy was used comparing the importance of the clinical history and lesion description in interpretation of cytologic findings with the patient history and the physical examination findings in providing a clinical diagnosis. The veterinary pathologist is trained to describe what he or she sees on the slide just as the clinician is trained to describe what he or she finds on physical examination. The comments that accompany the diagnosis and interpretation are used to incorporate the clinical findings and lesion description in support of a definitive diagnosis or to develop a differential diagnosis with a recommendation for further evaluation.

Many cytologists initially review cytologic preparations before reading the source or clinical history. This approach reinforces good descriptive skills. Additional knowledge regarding the clinical history and lesion description allows the pathologist to refine the evaluation of cells or stroma that should or should not be present. The nature of the lesion can have an impact on the definitive nature of a cytologic diagnosis. The cytologic characteristics of some neoplastic processes can be bland. Their behavior may be more aggressive than their individual cell's morphologic characteristics indicate, depending on the site or, in some cases, the species. An example of this is thyroid neoplasia in the dog and cat. Although the uniform nondescript epithelial cells obtained on aspiration of a canine thyroid neoplasm are morphologically similar to those aspirated from a feline thyroid nodule, in more than 95% of cases, they indicate an aggressive malignant neoplasm. If the clinical history indicates a well-circumscribed non-fixed mass in the area of the thyroid of a dog, the cytologic diagnosis might be "thyroid neoplasia," with the comment that thyroid neoplasia is usually aggressive in this species. If the lesion description provided indicates that the mass is fixed to the deep tissues and involves major vessels in the area of the jugular furrow, a more definitive diagnosis of "thyroid carcinoma" may be possible.

Specifying the method of collection and source is also important in the full evaluation of a cytologic sample. If the sample is obtained by a blind percutaneous procedure versus an ultrasound-guided aspirate, the cytologist may be more conservative in the interpretation if he or she cannot confirm the tissue identity. Specification of an exact source is necessary. The ambiguity of certain terms is often surprising. For instance, the term *cervical* can mean the neck area or the cervix, and abdomen and thorax can mean in or on the abdomen or thorax. Specific terms should be used to describe complex anatomic structures, such as the eye, lip, digit, and ear. General anatomic language, such as the oral cavity, muzzle, and face or head, should be avoided.

The pathologist's responsibility is to provide a cytology report that allows the clinician to make appropriate decisions. The elements of a cytology report are a well-organized detailed description, a cytologic diagnosis or interpretation, and comments necessary to qualify the diagnosis or interpretation. Within the description, the pathologist should indicate the quality of the preparation, including whether there are sufficient intact cells for evaluation and whether the sample is hemodiluted. A precise description of the cellular components can assist the clinician in discussing cases with other veterinary specialists, such as oncologists. The comments that accompany the diagnosis or interpretation should provide an indication of the degree of confidence if terms like *suspect*, *possible*, or *probable* are used. A differential diagnosis should be provided in cases in which a definitive diagnosis is not possible. Recommendations for additional testing can assist in better defining the cytologic findings.

CONFLICT RESOLUTION

There are times when there is discordance between cytologic and histologic diagnoses that may result in conflict between the clinician and the clinical pathologist. Conflict resolution is easiest when the lines of communication between the involved parties are open. A prompt discussion between the clinician and pathologist before additional diagnostics or clinical treatment decisions are made is essential when there is a question concerning the cytologic diagnosis. Clinicians should feel free to request a second-opinion evaluation in any case in which the cytologic diagnosis does not correlate with the clinical findings. Pathologists should accept requests for second opinions as part of their job. In fact, in many reference and academic clinical laboratories, in-house second opinions on difficult cytology samples are routinely performed.

As a professional courtesy, it is appropriate for the clinician to discuss the request for a second opinion and the reason for the request with the original pathologist. The conflict may be resolved with this step alone, especially if there is additional information that has an impact on the original interpretation. If the histopathology and cytology were done at the same laboratory, having them reviewed together may assist in determining the basis for the discordance; if they were done at separate laboratories, a discussion between the clinical pathologist and anatomic pathologist can be beneficial. A good cytologic preparation may be more useful than certain types of biopsies (ie, core or small wedge biopsies of a complex lesion). The prompt attention to issues concerning discordant diagnostic tests can lead to a more appropriate cytologic or histopathologic diagnosis, which, in turn, directs additional testing and an updated clinical diagnosis and treatment plan.

The recommended steps to take when there is a conflict between a cytologic diagnosis and the clinical findings or a subsequent histologic diagnosis are based on reviewing the case for errors in sample handling and communication: (1) confirm that an adequate and appropriate sample was submitted, (2) confirm that the sample was properly labeled, (3) request re-examination by the pathologist with communication of all pertinent background information, (4) determine if the sample submitted was representative, (5) request a second opinion from a pathologist, (6) reassess the clinical impression, (7) request a second opinion from a clinician, and (8) determine if the case may be an atypical presentation or a case with multiple disease processes.

CLINICAL CASES
Case 1: Hepatocellular Carcinoma Metastatic to Skin
A fine-needle aspirate of a "ventral abdominal mass" from a 10-year-old neutered female Domestic Shorthair cat was submitted for evaluation. The cytologic preparation consisted of sheets and clusters of anaplastic epithelial cells with pigment consistent with bile (Fig. 1). The cytologic diagnosis was hepatocellular carcinoma. The source of the sample was confirmed by the clinical pathologist because of the unusual diagnosis for a subcutaneous mass. Additional history indicated that a liver tumor had been removed a few months previously with no histopathologic evaluation. A subsequent excisional biopsy of the cutaneous mass was performed, and a histologic diagnosis of perianal adenocarcinoma was made (Fig. 2). To address the discordance, the clinical pathologist consulted with the histopathologist and provided the additional clinical history. After review of the histologic sections, the histologic diagnosis was revised to metastatic hepatic adenocarcinoma. A confounding factor resulting in the discordant diagnoses was the lack of bile pigment in the histologic sections. The epithelial cells of the perianal glands are remarkably similar to hepatocytes (hence, the alternate histologic diagnosis of hepatoid adenoma or adenocarcinoma for perianal gland tumors). The major points illustrated by this case are the necessity of a complete history for cytology and histopathology and the appropriate communication between all three individuals involved in the case.

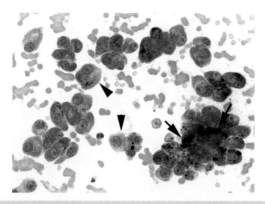

Fig. 1. Case 1. Fine-needle aspirate from the cutaneous nodule. The nucleated cells have uniform single round nuclei and abundant lightly basophilic cytoplasm (*arrowheads*) with intra- and extracellular dark pigment (*arrows*) consistent with bile (Wright's Giemsa stain, original magnification ×600).

Case 2: Well-Differentiated Tubuloacinar Nasal Adenocarcinoma

An impression preparation of a nasal biopsy from a 13-year-old neutered male Siamese cat was submitted with a clinical history of 2.5-year duration of a "runny nose" and 6 months of wheezing that was partially responsive to antibiotics. The cytologic description indicated sheets of homogeneous epithelial cells with plasma cells, lymphocytes, neutrophils, and bacteria. The cytologic diagnosis was epithelial hyperplasia with lymphoid aggregates, plasmacytosis, and secondary septic suppurative inflammation. The primary differential diagnosis was lymphoplasmacytic rhinitis (Figs. 3 and 4). The history provided for the biopsy specimen was chronic sinusitis, irritation, and inflammation. The

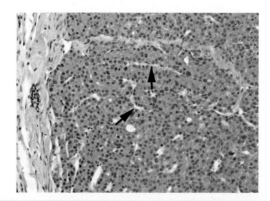

Fig. 2. Case 1. Histologic section of the cutaneous nodule. Note the epithelial cells with similar round nuclei and abundant eosinophilic cytoplasm forming linear rows with small sinusoid-like spaces (*arrows*) (hematoxylin-eosin stain, original magnification ×400).

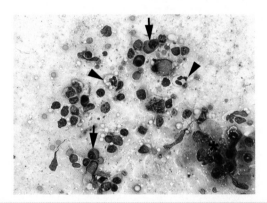

Fig. 3. Case 2. Impression preparation of the nasal biopsy. Note the mixed inflammatory cells, including neutrophils (*arrowheads*) and plasma cells (*arrows*). A cluster of respiratory epithelial cells is located in the lower right corner (*) (Wright's Giemsa stain, original magnification ×600).

histopathologic diagnosis was well-differentiated tubuloacinar nasal adenocarcinoma with a comment of "mild anisocytosis and anisokaryosis are seen" (Figs. 5 and 6). To address the discordant diagnoses, the cytology slides were reviewed and mild to moderate atypia was noted in the cytologic preparation. The case records contained a report for CT examination of the lesion that indicated a mass "extending through the bone around the eye invading the cribriform plate." This case is an excellent example of several issues: incomplete history, concurrent inflammation and sepsis confounding the interpretation of atypical epithelial cells, possible sample bias (with imprint preparations, only the surface cells are shed onto the slide), the conservative

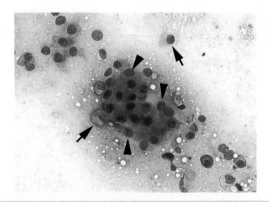

Fig. 4. Case 2. Impression preparation of the nasal biopsy. Note the relatively uniform epithelial nuclei (*arrowheads*) within the cluster of respiratory epithelial cells. The arrows denote plasma cells (Wright's Giemsa stain, original magnification ×600).

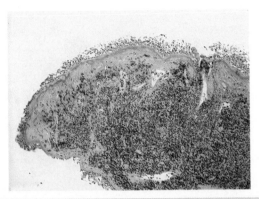

Fig. 5. Case 2. Histologic section of the nasal turbinate tissue. Note the submucosal proliferation of epithelial cells with small, round, deeply basophilic nuclei that occasionally form small circular (acinar-like) structures. The overlying respiratory epithelium is intact (hematoxylin-eosin stain, original magnification ×100).

nature of clinical pathologists in diagnosing neoplasia when there is significant inflammation and insufficient cellular pleomorphism to support a diagnosis of malignancy, and the necessity for tissue architecture in the diagnosis of well-differentiated neoplasia. A good history and lesion description do not change the objective evaluation of a slide or the differential list provided for the cytologic findings; they do change the subjective interpretation in the comments and the priority of the individual diagnoses on that list, however. With the clinical history of an invasive and destructive mass found on CT examination, the clinical pathologist might have included well-differentiated sinonasal adenocarcinoma as a primary differential diagnosis instead of hyperplasia, with the indication

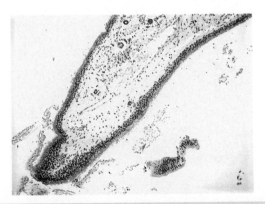

Fig. 6. Case 2. Histologic section of an area of the nasal biopsy unaffected by the neoplastic process. Note the intact respiratory epithelium overlying a mildly inflamed submucosa with no evidence of neoplasia evident (hematoxylin-eosin stain, original magnification ×100).

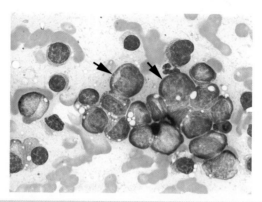

Fig. 7. Case 3. Fine-needle aspirate of the liver. The arrows indicate large lymphocytes with fine chromatin and a small to moderate amount of lightly basophilic cytoplasm (Wright's Giemsa stain, original magnification ×1000).

that histopathology would be necessary to rule out hyperplasia in response to the inflammation completely.

Case 3: Hepatic Lymphoma

A fine-needle aspirate of the liver from an 11-year-old neutered male Viszla was submitted for cytologic examination. The dog was previously diagnosed with protein-losing enteropathy and was currently receiving corticosteroid treatment. A CBC showed leukopenia (3,800 cells/μL), mild anemia (32% PCV), and thrombocytopenia (37,000 cells/μL). A clinical chemistry profile showed hypoalbuminemia (1.5 g/dL), elevated liver enzymes (alkaline phosphatase

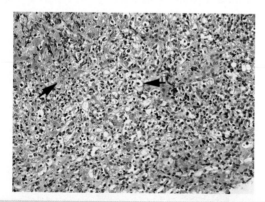

Fig. 8. Case 3. Histologic section of the liver biopsy. The left arrow indicates a remnant hepatocyte with moderately abundant eosinophilic cytoplasm. The right arrow indicates a large lymphocyte with clear cytoplasm. Note the difference in cellular detail between the cytologic preparation and the histologic section in this case (hematoxylin-eosin stain, original magnification ×400).

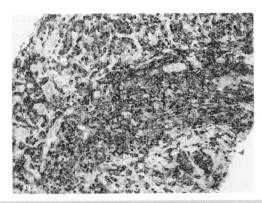

Fig. 9. Case 3. Immunohistochemical stain for CD3, a T-lymphocyte marker. The cytoplasm of the T cells stains reddish brown (hematoxylin counterstain, original magnification ×200).

[ALP] = 1659 U/L, alanine aminotransferase [ALT] = 569 U/L), and hyperbilirubinemia (2.9 mg/dL). A clotting profile showed prolonged prothrombin time (PT) and increased fibrin degradation products. Abdominal ultrasound examination revealed hepatosplenomegaly with hypoechoic nodules in the liver. The cytologic diagnosis was lymphoma based on finding many large lymphocytes intermixed with normal-appearing hepatocytes (Fig. 7). A subsequent core biopsy of the liver was submitted for histopathology, with a history of elevated liver enzymes, hypoproteinemia, pancytopenia, splenomegaly, and protein-losing enteropathy. The histopathologic diagnosis was hepatocellular carcinoma (Fig. 8). Because of the disparate results, the attending veterinarian requested a review of the histology slides by a clinical pathologist and the original case pathologist and a second pathologist. Immunohistochemical stains for

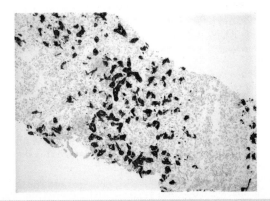

Fig. 10. Case 3. Immunohistochemical stain for cytokeratin, an epithelial cell marker. The cytoplasm of the residual hepatocytes stains reddish brown (hematoxylin counterstain, original magnification ×100).

cytokeratin (epithelial cell marker) and CD3 (T-cell marker) were performed to evaluate the cell populations. Most of the large neoplastic cells were identified as T cells by strong positive staining for CD3 (Fig. 9). The residual hepatocytes were strongly positive for cytokeratin (Fig. 10). The histologic diagnosis was revised to hepatic lymphoma. The primary point illustrated in this case is the difficulty in histologic interpretation of small needle biopsies that hinder sample orientation and often have "crush" artifact, compounded by an incomplete history that did not include the ultrasound findings or the cytologic diagnosis. In instances such as this, cytology often allows better individual cell evaluation than histopathology.

SUMMARY

Cytology is a valuable diagnostic tool in veterinary medicine. A review of the literature indicates its utility in evaluation of specific lesions. The information obtained from cytology is greatly enhanced by a good understanding of its advantages and disadvantages and an open and interactive relationship between clinicians and pathologists. Critical selection of appropriate lesions, good sampling technique, quality sample handling, and provision of a complete clinical history and lesion description enhance the utility of the information returned to the clinician by the pathologist. A good cytologic diagnosis is a team effort.

References

[1] Aitken ML, Patnaik AK. Comparison of needle-core (Trucut) biopsy and surgical biopsy for the diagnosis of cutaneous and subcutaneous masses: a prospective study of 51 cases (November 1997-August 1998). J Am Anim Hosp Assoc 2000;36(2):153–7.

[2] Willard MD, Jergens AE, Duncan RB, et al. Interobserver variation among histopathologic evaluations of intestinal tissues from dogs and cats [see comment]. J Am Vet Med Assoc 2002;220(8):1177–82.

[3] Willard MD, Lovering SL, Cohen ND, et al. Quality of tissue specimens obtained endoscopically from the duodenum of dogs and cats. J Am Vet Med Assoc 2001;219(4):474–9.

[4] Cohen M, Bohling MW, Wright JC, et al. Evaluation of sensitivity and specificity of cytologic examination: 269 cases (1999–2000). J Am Vet Med Assoc 2003;222(7):964–7.

[5] Eich CS, Whitehair JG, Moroff SD, et al. The accuracy of intraoperative cytopathological diagnosis compared with conventional histopathological diagnosis. J Am Anim Hosp Assoc 2000;36(1):16–8.

[6] Ghisleni G, Roccabianca P, Ceruti R, et al. Correlation between fine-needle aspiration cytology and histopathology in the evaluation of cutaneous and subcutaneous masses from dogs and cats. Vet Clin Pathol 2006;35(1):24–30.

[7] Twomey LN, Alleman AR. Cytodiagnosis of feline lymphoma. Comp Cont Ed Prac Vet 2005;27:17–32.

[8] Langenbach A, McManus PM, Hendrick MJ, et al. Sensitivity and specificity of methods of assessing the regional lymph nodes for evidence of metastasis in dogs and cats with solid tumors. J Am Vet Med Assoc 2001;218(9):1424–8.

[9] Williams LE, Packer RA. Association between lymph node size and metastasis in dogs with oral malignant melanoma: 100 cases (1987–2001). J Am Vet Med Assoc 2003;222(9):1234–6.

[10] Powe JR, Canfield PJ, Martin PA. Evaluation of the cytologic diagnosis of canine prostatic disorders. Vet Clin Pathol 2004;33(3):150–4.

[11] Wood EF, O'Brien RT, Young KM. Ultrasound-guided fine-needle aspiration of focal parenchymal lesions of the lung in dogs and cats. J Vet Intern Med 1998;12(5):338–42.

[12] DeBerry JD, Norris CR, Samii VF, et al. Correlation between fine-needle aspiration cytopathology and histopathology of the lung in dogs and cats. J Am Anim Hosp Assoc 2002;38(4):327–36.

[13] Caniatti M, Roccabianca P, Ghisleni G, et al. Evaluation of brush cytology in the diagnosis of chronic intranasal disease in cats. J Small Anim Pract 1998;39(2):73–7 [erratum appears in J Small Anim Pract 1998;39(4):202].

[14] Jergens AE, Andreasen CB, Hagemoser WA, et al. Cytologic examination of exfoliative specimens obtained during endoscopy for diagnosis of gastrointestinal tract disease in dogs and cats. J Am Vet Med Assoc 1998;213(12):1755–9.

[15] Jergens AE, Andreasen CB, Miles KG. Gastrointestinal endoscopic exfoliative cytology: techniques and clinical application. Comp Cont Ed Prac Vet 2000;22:941–52.

[16] Bennett PF, Hahn KA, Toal RL, et al. Ultrasonographic and cytopathological diagnosis of exocrine pancreatic carcinoma in the dog and cat. J Am Anim Hosp Assoc 2001;37(5): 466–73.

[17] Wang KY, Panciera DL, Al-Rukibat RK, et al. Accuracy of ultrasound-guided fine-needle aspiration of the liver and cytologic findings in dogs and cats: 97 cases (1990-2000). J Am Vet Med Assoc 2004;224(1):75–8.

[18] Roth L. Comparison of liver cytology and biopsy diagnosis in dogs and cats: 56 cases. Vet Clin Pathol 2001;30(1):35–8.

[19] Weiss DJ, Blauvelt M, Aird B. Cytologic evaluation of inflammation in canine liver aspirates. Vet Clin Pathol 2001;30(4):193–6.

[20] Cole TL, Center SA, Flood SN, et al. Diagnostic comparison of needle and wedge biopsy specimens of the liver in dogs and cats. J Am Vet Med Assoc 2002;220(10):1483–90.

[21] Stockhaus C, Van Den Ingh T, Rothuizen J, et al. A multistep approach in the cytologic evaluation of liver biopsy samples of dogs with hepatic diseases. Vet Pathol 2004;41(5): 461–70.

[22] Stockhaus C, Teske E, Van Den Ingh T, et al. The influence of age on the cytology of the liver in healthy dogs. Vet Pathol 2002;39(1):154–8.

[23] Higgins RJ, LeCouteur RA, Vernau KM, et al. Granular cell tumor of the canine central nervous system: two cases. Vet Pathol 2001;38(6):620–7.

[24] Long SN, Anderson TJ, Long FH, et al. Evaluation of rapid staining techniques for cytologic diagnosis of intracranial lesions. Am J Vet Res 2002;63(3):381–6.

[25] Platt SR, Alleman AR, Lanz OI, et al. Comparison of fine-needle aspiration and surgical-tissue biopsy in the diagnosis of canine brain tumors. Vet Surg 2002;31(1):65–9.

[26] Vernau KM, Higgins RJ, Bollen AW, et al. Primary canine and feline nervous system tumors: intraoperative diagnosis using the smear technique. Vet Pathol 2001;38(1):47–57.

[27] Zimmerman KL, Bender HS, Boon GD, et al. A comparison of the cytologic and histologic features of meningiomas in four dogs. Vet Clin Pathol 2000;29:29–34.

[28] Vignoli M, Ohlerth S, Rossi F, et al. Computed tomography-guided fine-needle aspiration and tissue-core biopsy of bone lesions in small animals. Vet Radiol Ultrasound 2004;45(2):125–30.

[29] Samii VF, Nyland TG, Werner LL, et al. Ultrasound-guided fine-needle aspiration biopsy of bone lesions: a preliminary report. Vet Radiol Ultrasound 1999;40(1):82–6.

[30] Reinhardt S, Stockhaus C, Teske E, et al. Assessment of cytological criteria for diagnosing osteosarcoma in dogs. J Small Anim Pract 2005;46(2):65–70.

[31] Hirschberger J, DeNicola DB, Hemanns W, et al. Sensitivity and specificity of cytologic evaluation in the diagnosis of neoplasia in body fluids from dogs and cats. Vet Clin Path 1999;28(4):1142–6.

[32] Costello MF, Drobatz KJ, Aronson LR, et al. Underlying cause, pathophysiologic abnormalities, and response to treatment in cats with septic peritonitis: 51 cases (1990–2001). J Am Vet Med Assoc 2004;225(6):897–902.

[33] Gibson NR, Carmicheal A, Li A, et al. Value of direct smears of synovial fluid in the diagnosis of canine joint disease. Vet Rec 1999;144(17):463–5.

[34] Meinkoth JH, Cowell RL. Sample collection and preparation in cytology: increasing diagnostic yield. Vet Clin North Am Small Anim Pract 2002;32(6):1187–207.

[35] Allen SW, Prasse KW, Mahaffey EA. Cytologic differentiation of benign from malignant canine mammary tumors. Vet Pathol 1986;23(6):649–55.

[36] Banin E, Brady KM, Greenberg EP. Chelator-induced dispersal and killing of Pseudomonas aeruginosa cells in a biofilm. Appl Environ Microbiol 2006;72(3):2064–9.

Vet Clin Small Anim 37 (2007) 373–392

VETERINARY CLINICS
SMALL ANIMAL PRACTICE

Fungal Diagnostics: Current Techniques and Future Trends

Sharon M. Dial, DVM, PhD

Department of Veterinary Science and Microbiology, Arizona Veterinary Diagnostic Laboratory, University of Arizona, 2831 North Freeway, Tucson, AZ 85705, USA

Fungal diseases are the great impersonators of human and veterinary medicine. The fungal agents that cause clinical disease can affect any organ system and present a wide spectrum of clinical and clinicopathologic signs. As with any disease process, the recognition of fungal disease requires that the etiologic agent be included in the initial differential diagnosis. The challenge does not stop there; if fungal disease is suspected, the options for a definitive diagnosis have historically been somewhat limited. The traditional methods for diagnosis of the various mycoses are based on detection of a serologic response to an agent, identification of an agent in cytologic or histopathologic specimens, or culture of the offending organism. The interpretation of fungal serologic testing is not straightforward; the available tests have variable sensitivity and specificity. In contrast, the specificity of cytology, histopathology, and culture approaches 100% depending on the expertise of the pathologist and laboratory, whereas the sensitivity is low overall because of the marked variability in the number of organisms within lesions.

The traditional methods for diagnosis of fungal disease have served veterinary and human medicine well for decades. With the expanding knowledge of molecular biology methods for detection of species-specific DNA and RNA within clinical specimens however, the traditional methods are being supported by new molecular techniques. The transition of polymerase chain reaction (PCR)–based amplification and sequencing of fungal DNA from the research laboratory to the diagnostic laboratory has occurred, with a few veterinary laboratories offering PCR-based tests with or without sequencing. Routine histologic methods are being enhanced by the development of specific immunohistochemical staining techniques that allow species identification in formalin-fixed paraffin-embedded tissues. These techniques are not going to replace the traditional methodologies in the near future, and perhaps never. They should greatly improve the identification of a class of agents that is often elusive, however. The need for species identification of the mycelial fungi is

E-mail address: sdial@u.arizona.edu

0195-5616/07/$ – see front matter
doi:10.1016/j.cvsm.2006.11.002

likely to drive the development of newer and, possibly, more species-directed antifungal therapeutics. A global approach to the diagnosis of fungal disease that correlates clinical signs as well as physical examination, clinical pathology, and histopathology findings with serology, culture, and the newer immunohistochemical and molecular techniques, where available, is the best approach to optimize the identification of the underlying agent.

CLINICAL PRESENTATION

Fungal agents have a remarkably varied repertoire of clinical signs: primary skin disease, single to multiple subcutaneous masses, mass lesions within body cavities, disseminated disease with multiple organ dysfunction, and disseminated disease that presents as single-organ dysfunction or as a cause of sudden death. Coccidioidomycosis, for example, can present with any of these scenarios. Coccidioidomycosis involving the heart and pericardium in the dog can be a final event in disseminated disease, resulting in sudden collapse and death with no prior indication of disease [1]. The fungal diseases can be divided into primary pathogens (ie, *Blastomyces*, *Histoplasma*, *Coccidioides*, *Cryptococcus*) and opportunistic pathogens (ie, *Aspergillus*, *Cladosporium*, *Conidiobolus*, *Basidiobolus*). The opportunistic pathogens include a large number of saprophytic soil fungi that cause disease when introduced into the tissues by focal trauma. They often present as a single subcutaneous mass or mycotic granuloma. With minimal tendency for disseminated disease. When dissemination of the opportunistic pathogens occurs, it is often associated with decreased immunocompetence.

There is some degree of "typical" presentation with several fungal agents: coccidioidomycosis, histoplasmosis, and blastomycosis are all primary pulmonary pathogens. Histoplasmosis is also associated with the gastrointestinal tract, whereas this organ system is rarely affected in coccidioidomycosis or blastomycosis. In turn, *Coccidioides* spp are more likely to disseminate to bone. Knowing the common presentations of each of the primary fungal agents keeps them at the forefront of a differential diagnosis. Knowing the talent these infectious agents have to mimic many diseases keeps them in the back of the clinician's mind to be pulled forth when there is an inappropriate response to therapy in a difficult case.

CLINICAL PATHOLOGY

Because of the diversity of organ systems that may become involved in disseminated fungal disease, there are no "typical" peripheral blood or serum chemistry changes associated with any fungal agent. Evidence of chronic inflammation, such as leukocytosis with a significant monocytosis or polyclonal hypergammaglobulinemia with increased inflammatory proteins with or without hypoalbuminemia, would support the suspicion of fungal disease. Because of the chronic nature of most fungal infections, a significant left shift to band neutrophils is not common. Nevertheless, these are largely nonspecific changes that can be seen with many inflammatory lesions. Peripheral eosinophilia is not a common finding with fungal disease, even though eosinophils are often a significant component of the tissue inflammatory response to fungal elements. Anemia of chronic disease is common with any chronic inflammatory disease, as is mild hypoalbuminemia. Hypercalcemia has been associated with granulomatous disease in human and veterinary medicine, with a specific association with histoplasmosis [2,3], blastomycosis [4,5], cryptococcosis [6,7], pneumocystosis [8–10], candidiasis [11], and coccidioidomycosis [6,12–14]. The mechanism for hypercalcemia has been shown to be increased circulating 1,25-dihydroxyvitamin D in several human cases and is more often associated with the granulomatous inflammatory process than with the organism [7,15]. In human beings, significant hypercalcemia is also seen with sarcoidosis, berylliosis, and tuberculosis [16]. Macrophages within these lesions interfere with the normal regulation of 1,25-dihydroxyvitamin D; hypercalcemia resolves when the granulomatous inflammatory response abates [16].

Cytology is one of the most useful clinical pathology techniques for identification of fungal disease. The cytologic characteristics of most fungal pathogens are well described in several veterinary textbooks [17,18] and are not reiterated in this article. Cytologic examination of body cavity fluids, skin, soft tissue masses and internal organ aspirates, transtracheal or bronchoalveolar lavage fluids, urine, and feces can provide a definitive diagnosis of fungal disease if the fungal organism is present in sufficient numbers within the tissues (Figs. 1 and 2). Urine and feces are often overlooked as cytologic samples. *Histoplasma capsulatum, Prototheca zopfii,* and *Cryptococcus neoformans* [19] can be found on fecal cytology if there is gastrointestinal involvement in disseminated disease or as a primary gastrointestinal pathogen. *Aspergillus* spp [20] and *Candida* spp [21] have been identified by cytology or culture of urine in cases of disseminated disease or primary urinary disease. Although the specificity of these techniques is high, the sensitivity varies considerably. The major advantage of cytology is its convenience and speed. The proficiency of the individual evaluating

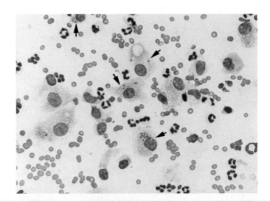

Fig. 1. Lung aspirate from a cat. Numerous large epithelioid macrophages and nondegenerate neutrophils are present. Macrophages containing small 1- to 2-μm yeast organisms are indicated by the arrows (Wright's Giemsa stain, original magnification ×400).

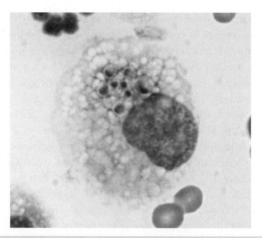

Fig. 2. Higher magnification of a macrophage illustrates the typical cytologic appearance of *Histoplasma capsulatum*. The yeast organisms have a dense basophilic nucleus and a clear "halo" or pseudocapsule (Wright's Giemsa stain, original magnification ×1000).

the slide is the primary variable in using cytology in the clinical setting. A good-quality clean cytologic stain is necessary. Wright's Giemsa and modified Wright's Giemsa stains adequately stain most fungal organisms within cytologic preparations. There are a few exceptions, such as the oomycetes (unique fungus-like pathogens) *Pythium* and *Lagenidium*, which have low affinity for most cytologic and histologic stains. Organisms that do not stain well appear as negatively stained elements that are easily overlooked (Fig. 3). India ink is often recommended for the identification of cryptococcal species because it shows the mucin capsule of this organism nicely. In practice, the proteinaceous

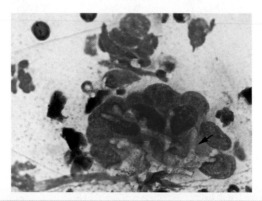

Fig. 3. Aspirate of a thoracic mass from a dog. The arrow indicates negatively staining mycelia within a multinucleate giant cell (Wright's Giemsa stain, original magnification ×1000).

background and surrounding inflammatory cells are usually just as useful for demonstrating the capsule and are less prone to artifact (Fig. 4). In addition, the lack of a capsule does not rule out *Cryptococcus* spp, because there are acapsular strains that can be difficult to differentiate from *Candida* spp [22]. When examining a cytologic preparation, it is important to keep in mind that fungi can occasionally present with atypical morphology. *Coccidioides* spp spherules can be easily confused with blastomycosis if they are small and in close juxtaposition (Fig. 5). In addition, rarely, only endospores from the ruptured spherules may be present and easily overlooked or confused with other agents [23]. Fig. 6 illustrates a case of coccidioidomycosis with rare small spherules and large numbers of free endospores, some of which could be confused with agents like *Prototheca* spp. Because many of the deep fungal infections have regional distributions, travel history can be especially important when evaluating atypical presentations for these diseases.

In many cases, the most useful aspect of a cytologic preparation is the identification of the typical inflammatory response to fungal agents: granulomatous to pyogranulomatous inflammation with or without eosinophils, mast cells, multinucleate giant cells, and reactive fibrocytes (Fig. 7). Fungal disease should be strongly suspected when this type of inflammatory response is identified regardless of whether or not an etiologic agent is seen. Because mixed bacterial and fungal infections do occur, septic inflammatory lesions that are unresponsive to appropriate medical therapy should be investigated further to rule out underlying mycotic disease. In human beings, 25% of nonresponsive "bacterial" pneumonias are actually fungal, with secondary bacterial disease [24]. The identification of a bacterial agent does not rule out a fungal component. This is especially true in cytology of the nasal cavity, in which primary fungal disease is often associated with secondary bacterial infection. With the mycelial

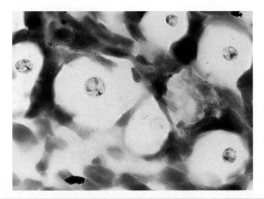

Fig. 4. Aspirate of a subcutaneous nodule from a cat. The large clear capsule of *Cryptococcus neoformans* is well defined by the adjacent erythrocytes. Note the basophilic cytoplasm with an eccentrically placed nucleus typically seen in this organism (Wright's Giemsa stain, original magnification ×1000).

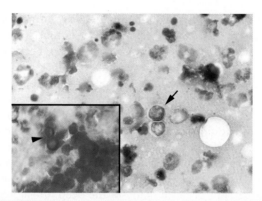

Fig. 5. Aspirate of a draining cutaneous lesion from a dog. Two small spherules of *Cocci-dioides* spp (*arrow*) in close association can easily mimic the yeast forms of *Blastomyces dermatitidis*. Rare large spherules and free endospores were seen throughout the preparation to assist in identifying the organism as *Coccidioides* spp. (*Inset*) Budding *B dermatitides* (*arrow-head*) (Wright's Giemsa stain, original magnification ×400).

fungi, such as *Aspergillus* spp, cytologic characteristics cannot definitively iden-tify the species and culture is need for final identification. The morphologic characterization of fungi growing in tissue can be significantly different from the morphology of the fungi when grown on fungal media. Structures like chlamydospores (Fig. 8) are commonly formed in tissues by many fungal agents that do not readily form these structures when cultured.

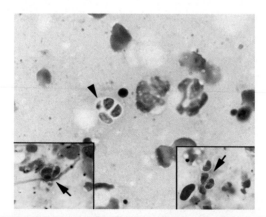

Fig. 6. Aspirate of a draining cutaneous lesion in a dog (same sample as in Fig. 5). In this small aggregate of *Coccidioides* spp, endospores with prominent septa between the individual endospores resemble a *Prototheca zopfii* organism (*arrowhead*). This was the predominant form of the organism seen in this preparation. Only rare spherules were found on close examination of all slides submitted. (*Insets*) *P zopfii* (*arrows*) (Wright's Giemsa stain, original magnification ×1000).

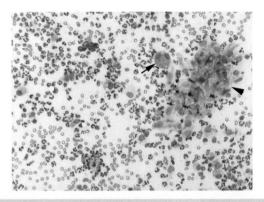

Fig. 7. Lung aspirate from a dog. Pyogranulomatous inflammation with multinucleate giant cells (*arrow*) and aggregates of fibroblasts (*arrowhead*) is typical of the inflammatory response seen in many fungal lesions. *Coccidioides* spp was cultured from pleural fluid submitted with this aspirate (Wright's Giemsa stain, original magnification ×200).

HISTOPATHOLOGY

The histologic diagnosis of fungal disease shares the same specificity and sensitivity as cytologic preparations. Again, the sensitivity depends greatly on the number of organisms present in the tissue submitted. Fig. 9 illustrates a single spherule of *Coccidioides* spp found on 1 of 10 step sections of a bone core biopsy. The original section evaluated by the pathologist had the typical inflammatory lesion for coccidioidal osteomyelitis that prompted collection of the additional sections to search for the organism. Sample size is often the determining factor in providing a histologic diagnosis. As with cytology, although no etiologic

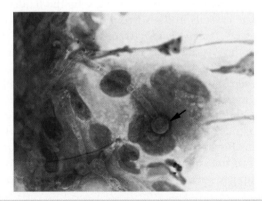

Fig. 8. Corneal scraping from a horse. The arrow indicates a terminal chlamydoconidium-like swelling at the end of a septate mycelium. These structures can be numerous or rare depending on the fugal species and, possibly, host factors that influence fungal growth within tissues (Wright's Giemsa stain, original magnification ×1000).

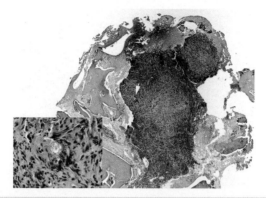

Fig. 9. Bone biopsy from a lytic and proliferative lesion on the distal femur of a dog. There is a large focus of pyogranulomatous inflammation with a single spherule of *Coccidioides* spp indicated by the arrow (hematoxylin-eosin stain, original magnification ×40). (*Inset*) Higher power view of spherule (hematoxylin-eosin stain, original magnification ×400).

agents are identified on routine stains, the characteristics of the inflammatory response often prompt application of special stains that may assist in finding fungal agents present in small numbers. Routine use of periodic acid–Shiff (PAS) and Gomori's methenamine silver (GMS) stains often confirms the suspicion of fungal disease. With the dimorphic fungi, such as *Coccidioides* spp, the histologic appearance of the tissue phase usually allows for species identification. This is not true for the mycelial fungal agents. Although there are characteristics that can assist in placing the fungal agent identified into broad groups of fungi (Zygomycetes, Hyalohyphomycetes, and Phaeohyphomycetes), there are no histologic features that are diagnostic for any of the mycelial pathogens. An exception to this rule may be the tendency for *Aspergillus niger* to form oxalate crystals in the surrounding tissue (Fig. 10) [25]. The two pathogenic oomycetes *Pythium insidiosum* and *Lagenidium* spp cannot be easily distinguished from the Zygomycetes in tissue and are difficult to isolate in culture [26]. Fungal pathogens are described based on pigmentation (dematiaceous fungi), degree of septation, and width and degree of parallelism of mycelia. From these characteristics, the pathologist can usually provide a list of possible etiologic agents. Although rare, dual infections with two fungal pathogens do occur. Fig. 11 illustrates a concurrent infection in a dog with *Coccidioides* spp and a dematiaceous fungus. The dog had an antemortem diagnosis of coccidioidomycosis but was unresponsive to antifungal therapy. As with the cytologic identification of fungal agents, culture is usually needed to make the final identification.

SEROLOGY

The use of serology in the diagnosis of fungal disease challenges the clinician's skills in interpretation of laboratory data. The first step in understanding

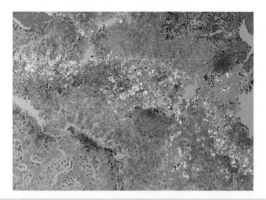

Fig. 10. Nasal biopsy from a dog. Large numbers of birefringent crystals consistent with calcium oxalate are present in association with a large fungal mat adherent to nasal turbinate tissue. Fugal culture had a heavy growth of *Aspergillus niger* (hematoxylin-eosin stain under polarized light, original magnification ×100).

serology is to be sure the methodology and its limitations are understood, including the sensitivity and specificity of individual tests. A firm understanding of these factors is necessary to use serology to its fullest capacity. This is especially true for fungal serology, because each serologic test for each agent has its problems. The difficulty in determining the true sensitivity of a serologic test for fungal disease is evident by the lack of references that can provide such data based on sufficiently large veterinary epidemiologic studies. Sensitivity

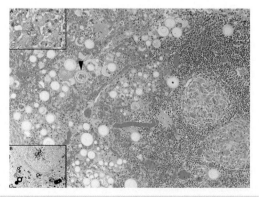

Fig. 11. Splenic tissue from a dog. Numerous viable (*arrowhead*) and empty (*asterisk*) spherules of *Coccidioides* spp and two small well-defined granulomas (*lower right corner*) are present (hematoxylin-eosin stain, original magnification ×100). (*Inset A*) Higher power view of a granuloma containing pigmented (dematiaceous) fungal hyphae (hematoxylin-eosin stain, original magnification ×400). (*Inset B*) GMS stain shows both types of fungi (*black*) present within the splenic tissue (original magnification ×100).

and specificity data for the serologic tests for blastomycosis [27], histoplasmosis [28], and cryptococcosis [29] have been reported. The specificity of fungal serologic tests can be more readily evaluated in the clinical and laboratory setting. Table 1 lists the currently available serologic tests for several fungal agents and their characteristics. Most of the fungal serologic tests currently in use in veterinary medicine detect the humoral (antibody) response to exposure. In contrast, tests that detect fungal antigens may provide a definitive diagnosis if the antigen test is sufficiently specific. The antigen-based latex agglutination test available for *C neoformans* is the most widely used antigen-based fungal serologic test. Additional enzyme-linked immunoassays (EIAs) for antigenemia or antigenuria have been developed for the diagnosis of histoplasmosis [30] and aspergillosis [31] in human beings and for the diagnosis of blastomycosis [32] in dogs. As with any serologic test, cross-reactivity must be evaluated, because many fungal agents share structural antigens. The EIA test for *H capsulatum* can cross-react with several fungal agents, including *Paracoccidioides brasiliensis, Blastomyces dermatitidis, Coccidioides immitis*, and *Penicillium marneffei* [33]. Currently, antigen-based tests are available for *C neoformans, B dermatitidis*, and *Aspergillosis* spp [18].

With all antibody-based serologic tests, overinterpretation is a significant problem. Persistent titers after exposure with elimination of the agent are confounding factors in the accurate diagnosis of blastomycosis and coccidioidomycosis. Few serologic tests provide a definitive diagnosis. Positive serology should be considered evidence of exposure that supports the clinical findings. Paired serum samples (2–3 weeks apart) should be run concurrently. A four-fold increase or decrease in the titer is strong evidence of active disease. It is important to stress that the paired samples must be run at the same time because of the interassay variability of serologic tests. This necessitates saving a portion of the initial serum sample to be submitted with the second specimen. The exception may be the ELISA test for pythiosis. Using a 40% percent positive value compared with positive control serum run simultaneously with patient serum, Grooters and colleagues [34] showed 100% sensitivity and 100% specificity for this test comparing samples from clinically healthy dogs, dogs infected with *P insidiosum*, dogs with nonpythium fungal and protozoal disease, and dogs with noninfectious gastrointestinal disease. In addition, this serologic test can be used for postsurgical follow-up, with recrudescence of the disease resulting in increasing serum titers.

A single serologic test can often be misleading in the differentiation of fungal disease and other inflammatory and neoplastic diseases in regions with endemic fungal diseases. In a recent serologic survey of *Coccidioides* spp in the Southwest, positive agar gel immunodiffusion (AGID) titers as high as 1:16 were found in clinically normal dogs [35]. Complement fixation titers have been used in the past for *Coccidioides* spp serology. Unfortunately, up to 25% of canine serum samples are anticomplementary and cannot be titered with this method. As a result, most laboratories providing *Coccidioides* spp serology use the AGID test.

Table 1
Serologic tests available for selected fungal agents

	Blastomyces	Coccidioides	Cryptococcus	Histoplasma	Aspergillus	Pythium
Primary methodology	AGID	AGID	Antigen latex agglutination	AGID	AGID	ELISA
Sensitivity/ specificity	90%/90% [27]	Not known/>95%	90%–100%/ 97%–100% [29]	Poor sensitivity and specificity [28]	Not known	100%/100%
Cross-reactivity	Minimal	Minimal	Minimal	Blastomycosis, penicilliosis, coccidioidomycosis	Minimal	Minimal
Problems	Negative early, persistent titers confound interpretation	Negative in some disseminated cases, insufficient data to assess predictive value of titers, persistent titers confound interpretation	Minimal, test can be performed on serum, urine, or CSF and can be used to follow therapy	Large number of false-negative results, especially in early disease	False-negative results not uncommon	Minimal, titers can be used to follow therapy

Abbreviations: AGID, agar gel immunodiffusion; CSF, cerebrospinal fluid.

As with all diagnostic tests, the history, physical examination findings, and additional diagnostic test results are requisites for interpretation of positive or negative serology. The poor specificity of the available serologic tests for histoplasmosis essentially negates the value of serology for this disease. The increased use of immune-suppressive agents for treatment of neoplasia and immune-mediated disease provides fertile ground for an increase in fungal diseases in companion animals. This has been evident in human medicine and is likely to follow in veterinary medicine [36]. In these patients, an unresponsive immune system can lead to seronegative disease.

CULTURE

The "gold standard" for the specific identification of fungal disease is culture of the suspected organism from fluids or tissue. Again, sensitivity is the primary issue in depending on culture alone for diagnosis. The sensitivity for culture of *H capsulatum* in human pulmonary histoplasmosis ranges from 15% to 85% depending on the type of disease (ie, acute versus chronic disease) [37]. The probability of successful culture of fungal agents depends on several variables: concentration of fungal elements in the sample, sample integrity, culture requirements of the fungal agent, and expertise of the laboratory performing the culture.

Obtaining and submitting the appropriate sample for culture is the first and most important step. Providing the laboratory with a detailed history, accurate source, and clinical diagnosis can greatly enhance the potential for successful culture and identification of a fungal agent. Although culturettes are commonly used to submit samples for bacterial and fungal culture, they are not the method preferred by most microbiology laboratorians. Samples of body cavity fluids, urine, and exudates can be submitted in sterile serum collection tubes (red top) and concentrated at the laboratory to facilitate culture of the agents. Up to 10 mL of fluid is recommended. Urine is often overlooked as a sample for identification of disseminated fungal disease. *Cryptococcus* and *Aspergillus* fungal element have been recovered from urine samples in dogs with disseminated disease [20,21,38]. If the lesion is a mass, dermal, subcutaneous, or internal fresh tissue can be submitted in a sterile container for culture. It is often useful to submit formalin-fixed tissue for histopathology at the same time. Many fungal species grow slowly; identifying the organism in histologic sections often justifies retention of cultures for an extended period or prompts the use of enrichment media to facilitate successful identification of the agent. *P insidiosum*, an oomycete, is difficult to distinguish from Zygomycetes in tissue sections and requires specific handling to decrease the effect of bacterial overgrowth on the viability and growth of the organism [39]. Alerting the laboratory to the possibility of infection with this agent facilitates its growth and identification.

Identification of fungal agents in cultures requires patience. The cultures must mature and form characteristic fruiting bodies, conidia, or arthrospores to allow morphologic identification of the fungus. For some fungal species, specific media are needed to promote the production of the asexual stage and its characteristic morphology. In addition, certain species of fungi are sufficiently similar that growth characteristics on multiple media must be evaluated for definitive species identification [40].

The tissue phase of most pathogenic fungi poses little danger to those handling patients with active disease. The exception is the saprophytic yeast *Sporothrix schenckii*, which is a zoonotic disease agent that can be transmitted to individuals handling the patient if appropriate precautions are not taken. In contrast, once the agent has been isolated on microbiologic media and has formed spores or conidia, there is significant potential for inhalation by laboratory personnel. It is strongly advised that fungal culture (other than for dermatophytosis) be left to the diagnostic laboratory setting. All fungal cultures at the University of Arizona are sealed to limit exposure of laboratory personnel to potential infectious particles. The cultures are only opened for evaluation in a biocontainment hood, because aerosolization of the spores is easy when culture plates are opened. The fungus is treated with formalin before microscopic evaluation. Recognition and identification of fungal structures are much like cytology; the proficient individual is one who develops expertise through experience. All these factors speak to the wisdom of leaving fungal isolation and identification to the trained mycologist rather than attempting to have an in-house mycology laboratory.

IMMUNOHISTOCHEMISTRY

In the past decade, immunohistochemistry (IHC) has become a routine method for detection and specific identification of infectious agents within biopsy and necropsy tissues in veterinary medicine. Most of the agents identified by this method are bacterial, viral, and protozoal. There are increasing numbers of veterinary diagnostic laboratories offering IHC as a method to speciate fungal organisms within tissues submitted for routine histopathology, however. Currently, Michigan State University and Kansas State University diagnostic laboratories offer IHC tests for fungal diseases, including aspergillosis, blastomycosis, histoplasmosis, coccidioidomycosis, and candidiasis. Although reports in the veterinary literature are few at this time, as more laboratories develop IHC as a routine part of their diagnostic offering, its utility should become better documented. Thus far, IHC for the detection and identification of pseudomycetoma attributable to *Microsporum canis* [41] and for equine [42] and canine pythiosis [43] has been reported.

The principle of IHC is similar to that of an indirect ELISA on tissue sections. The sensitivity and specificity of an IHC stain largely depend on the primary antibody directed at the target antigen. Individual antibodies vary significantly in affinity for the target antigen and have different levels of cross-reactivity to associated or similar antigens. Individual laboratories must standardize and validate all IHC stains offered. The American Association of Veterinary Laboratory Diagnosticians Subcommittee on Immunohistochemistry has developed guidelines for IHC standardization. Although IHC can be used as a stand-alone test, in most cases, IHC and routine histopathology must be evaluated in tandem to provide the most information.

As with all diagnostic test procedures, the integrity of the sample is paramount for diagnosis. One factor that can adversely affect IHC staining is the length of time the tissue has been in formalin. Excessive cross-linking of antigen protein by formalin interferes with recognition of the antigen by the primary antibody in the IHC procedure. There is a broad range for the time of formalin exposure that results in significant interference with individual antibody-antigen interactions. If tissues have been held in formalin before submission for histopathologic examination, the duration of time in formalin should be included in the history. At most reference laboratories, tissues are processed within 24 hours after receipt of the sample.

There are numerous variables that must be defined within the laboratory setting for each IHC stain offered, including the type of tissue section pretreatment that might be needed to enhance affinity of the primary antibody to the antigen, length of primary antibody incubation, and type of detection system used. Such problems as nonspecific staining or high background staining can make interpretation of IHC stains difficult. Cross-reactivity must be evaluated with respect to similar agents. A good example of the cross-reactivity of antibodies to infectious agents is the bacillus Calmette-Guerin (BCG) polyclonal antibody directed against the cell wall component of *Mycobacterium bovis*. This antibody is strongly cross-reactive with several bacterial and nonbacterial infectious agents, including *B dermatitidis*, *Coccidioides* spp, *Cryptococcus* spp, *H capsulatum*, *Malassezia* spp, *Sporothrix* spp, *Pythium* spp, *Prototheca* spp, dermatophytes, and Phaeohyphomycetes [44,45]. The BCG antibody can be helpful in identification of fungi that do not stain well with traditional stains, such as GMS or PAS stains (Fig. 12), and as a "survey" stain for lesions that may have multiple etiologic agents present.

A major advantage of IHC over culture and purely molecular technologies is the visual identification of the organism within the context of the diseased tissue. Interpretation of culture without histologic visualization of fungal elements in the tissues can be difficult when opportunistic agents are involved, because many of these agents can be contaminants. Histologic evaluation may simply provide an inflammatory context that supports the possibility of fungal disease. The same is true for the molecular methods to be discussed. Finding *Aspergillus* DNA in a corneal scrapping sample is much stronger evidence of fungal keratitis when there is histologic or cytologic evidence of typical inflammation associated with fungal disease. An excellent Internet site to review the number of laboratories currently offering IHC for diagnosis of infectious disease is the IHC database developed and maintained at the South Dakota State University diagnostic laboratory [46].

MOLECULAR TECHNIQUES

Increasingly, clinicians in human and veterinary medicine are looking toward PCR-based diagnostic tests as routine. For the most part, development of

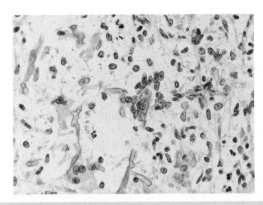

Fig. 12. Gastric mass from a dog. The broad variable-width mycelia of *Pythium insidiosum* (*brown*) stained with a polyclonal anti-*Mycobacterium bovis* BCG antibody. The dog was serologically positive by the ELISA method, and sections of the mass also stained positive for *P insidiosum* by IHC (polyclonal rabbit anti-*M bovis*, 1:1000; diaminobenzidine [DAB] substrate, Dako [Carpinteria, CA]; hematoxylin counterstain, original magnification ×1000).

molecular techniques in veterinary medicine has focused on bacterial and viral disease. Increasing numbers of reports concerning the use of these molecular tests in the more complex organisms, such as protozoa and fungi, have been surfacing in the human and veterinary literature, however. The explosion of PCR diagnostics currently available can be accessed on the Internet at a companion to the South Dakota State University diagnostic laboratory IHC site [47]. Currently, specific tests for *Candida* spp and *Blastomyces* spp and a "panfungal" PCR test are available for diagnostic testing. Techniques for fungal molecular diagnostics have been primarily used for plant pathogens [48]. The primary advantages of PCR-based molecular methods are sensitivity and, with the development of newer real-time PCR techniques, speed. The primary disadvantage is the quality control of diagnostic testing.

The use of molecular-based testing in the human medical setting is undergoing extensive evaluation to develop an appropriate method of quality control and standardization of methods [48–50]. Because of the sensitivity of these techniques, contamination of samples and the subsequent reporting of false-positive results is a major concern within the laboratory setting; diligent standard laboratory practices are required to ensure accurate results. In addition, biologic samples as compared with pure cultures can contain inhibitory substances that can cause false-negative results [48,51]. The "specific" primers used in PCR can be less than specific, with amplification of nontarget DNA resulting in results that are difficult to interpret.

All these issues aside, the continued development of standardized and tested protocols for the identification of fungal pathogens is likely to progress as the need for more precise and timely diagnosis is made evident by the clinician. The development of a PCR protocol for any agent is a three-step process: (1) design primers to identify a target segment of DNA specific for an agent, (2) optimize extraction of total DNA from a biologic sample, and (3) determine the optimum conditions for amplification of the target DNA by the primers.

There are several approaches to optimizing the outcome. Selection of target DNA with multiple copies within the genome can enhance the sensitivity. Nesting a reaction by performing two amplification processes using "universal" primers that target a class of organisms is another approach. In fungal diagnostics, the universal primers are the highly conserved internal transcribed spacer (ITS) regions of the ribosomal DNA that flank more species-specific 25S, 18S, and 5.8S ribosomal genes. By using two of the five known ITS regions as the initial reaction, the more specific primers for the 18S or 5.8S ribosomal gene can be "nested" to provide the needed specificity. Alternatively, the initial amplification product produced by the use of the ITS primers can be sequenced and then compared with the ever-expanding genomic databases available. Detection of *Aspergillus fumigatus* [52], *C neoformans* [53], *Pythium* and *Lagenidium* [54], and *H capsulatum* [55] from clinical samples using the 18S ribosomal DNA gene or ITS regions has been reported.

It is important to note that identification by DNA sequencing of the ITS or 18S DNA gene is not always definitive. The ability to identify a fungal organism depends on whether or not the DNA of the fungus in question has been previously sequenced and submitted to the genomic databases. Millar and colleagues [56] reported the potential misidentification of an unknown fungal culture as *C immitis* when identification was based on the 18S DNA sequence alone. The misidentification occurred because the 18S DNA sequence for *Chrysosporium keratinophilum* was not available in the genomic database and these two fungi have 99.4% sequence identity for the 18S region. The 5.8S DNA sequence was more specific, however; the clinical sample had 100% sequence identity with the published 5.8S DNA sequence of *C keratinophilum* and only 84.7% sequence identity with the published 5.8S DNA sequence of *C immitis*. This case suggests that fungal identification based on DNA sequencing should include at least two DNA regions for comparison.

Unlike identification of fungal agents in tissues, PCR-based methods are commonly used to confirm identification of fungi in culture. Because of the hazard to laboratory personnel when handling cultures after they have formed the morphologically specific asexual structures, DNA probes that can be used on immature cultures to identify the fungal agent have been developed. DNA probes are labeled, complimentary, single-stranded DNA segments specific for unique regions of fungal DNA, usually the ribosomal RNA gene. The principle of the test is similar to that of an ELISA-based test. The labeled single-stranded DNA probe is used in place of the labeled antibody and aligns with complementary DNA if present in the sample being tested. Gen-Probe (SanDiego, CA) has developed fungal identification kits for *Blastomyces*, *Coccidioides*, and *Histoplasma* using chemiluminescent-labeled DNA probes. These DNA probe based kits are likely to gain common use in most microbiology laboratories that routinely identify fungal pathogens.

Microarray technology often takes PCR methods to a higher utility. Using microarray technology in which probes specific for DNA from a range of infectious agents are fixed to small areas on a solid phase, such as a glass slide, clinical samples can be screened for multiple organisms simultaneously. This technique has been developed for clinical samples to screen for bacterial [57] and viral [58] antigens in human beings. Currently, microarray technology in mycology has focused on examination of the genome of specific pathogens for identification of genes related to pathogenicity [59] and determination of differential gene expression during saprophytic and parasitic growth phages [60]. As better understanding of the fungal pathogen genomes emerges, development of species-specific probes should allow microarray technology to be used for screening clinical samples in mycotic disease as well.

SUMMARY

The diagnosis of fungal disease is a challenge that requires diligent attention to history and clinical signs as well as an astute ability to interpret laboratory data. Because fungal disease can mimic other infectious and neoplastic diseases in clinical presentation, the clinician has to be aware of fungal diseases common locally as well as in other regions of the country. The traditional methods of fungal pathogen identification by cytology, histopathology, and culture and the use of serology to support exposure to specific agents have served the veterinarian for many decades and should continue to be useful for many more. Nevertheless, newer techniques are now available that provide additional methods to identify specific fungal pathogens in samples in which the traditional methods have failed. IHC can assist in speciating agents when fresh tissue is not available for culture, and PCR techniques can assist in identification of agents in samples containing small numbers of organisms. With the ongoing development of molecular techniques, new methods, such as microarrays, allow screening of clinical samples for multiple infectious agents and are likely to become as common as the traditional methods. All diagnostic test results must be interpreted within the context of the patient, however.

References

[1] Shubitz LF, Matz ME, Noon TH, et al. Constrictive pericarditis secondary to Coccidioides immitis infection in a dog. J Am Vet Med Assoc 2001;218(4):537–40.

[2] Weller RE, Dagle GE, Malaga CA, et al. Hypercalcemia and disseminated histoplasmosis in an owl monkey. J Med Primatol 1990;19(7):675–80.

[3] Hodges RD, Legendre AM, Adams LG, et al. Itraconazole for the treatment of histoplasmosis in cats. J Vet Intern Med 1994;8(6):409–13.

[4] Dow SW, Legendre AM, Stiff M, et al. Hypercalcemia associated with blastomycosis in dogs. J Am Vet Med Assoc 1986;188(7):706–9.

[5] Storms TN, Clyde VL, Munson L, et al. Blastomycosis in nondomestic felids. J Zoo Wildl Med 2003;34(3):231–8.

[6] Ali MY, Gopal KV, Llerena LA, et al. Hypercalcemia associated with infection by Cryptococcus neoformans and Coccidioides immitis. Am J Med Sci 1999;318(6):419–23.

[7] Wang IK, Shen TY, Lee KF, et al. Hypercalcemia and elevated serum 1,25-dihydroxyvitamin D in an end-stage renal disease patient with pulmonary cryptococcosis. Ren Fail 2004; 26(3):333–8.

[8] Hung YM. Pneumocystis carinii pneumonia with hypercalcemia and suppressed parathyroid hormone levels in a renal transplant patient. Transplantation 2006; 81(4):639.

[9] Krebs M, Watschinger B, Brunner C, et al. Pneumocystis carinii in a patient with hypercalcemia and renal failure secondary to sarcoidosis. Wien Klin Wochenschr 2002;114(17–18): 785–8.

[10] Chen WC, Chang SC, Wu TH, et al. Hypercalcemia in a renal transplant recipient suffering with Pneumocystis carinii pneumonia. Am J Kidney Dis 2002;39(2):1–5.

[11] Kantarjian HM, Saad MF, Estey EH, et al. Hypercalcemia in disseminated candidiasis. Am J Med 1983;74(4):721–4.

[12] Lee JC, Catanzaro A, Parthemore JG, et al. Hypercalcemia in disseminated coccidioidomycosis. N Engl J Med 1977;297(8):431–3.

[13] Parker MS, Dokoh S, Woolfenden JM, et al. Hypercalcemia in coccidioidomycosis. Am J Med 1984;76(2):341–4.

[14] Westphal SA. Disseminated coccidioidomycosis associated with hypercalcemia. Mayo Clin Proc 1998;73(9):893–4.

[15] Spindel SJ, Hamill RJ, Georghiou PR, et al. Case report: vitamin D-mediated hypercalcemia in fungal infections. Am J Med Sci 1995;310(2):71–6.

[16] Sharma OP. Hypercalcemia in granulomatous disorders: a clinical review. Curr Opin Pulm Med 2000;6(5):442–7.

[17] Cowell RL, Tyler RD, Meinkoth JH. Diagnostic cytology and hematology of the dog and cat. 2nd edition. St. Louis (MO): Mosby; 1999.

[18] Greene CE. Infectious diseases of the dog and cat. 3rd edition. St Louis (MO): Saunders Elsevier; 2006.

[19] Graves TK, Barger AM, Adams B, et al. Diagnosis of systemic cryptococcosis by fecal cytology in a dog. Vet Clin Pathol 2005;34(4):409–12.

[20] Bruchim Y, Elad D, Klainbart S. Disseminated aspergillosis in two doges in Israel. Mycoses 2006;49(2):130–3.

[21] Adamama-Moraitou KK, Paitaki CG, Rallis TS, et al. Aspergillus species cystitis in a cat. J Feline Med Surg 2001;3(1):31–4.

[22] Laurenson IF, Ross JD, Milne LJ. Microscopy and latex antigen negative cryptococcal meningitis. J Infect 1998;36(3):329–31.

[23] Beaudin S, Rich LJ, Meinkoth JH, et al. Draining skin lesion from a desert poodle. Vet Clin Pathol 2005;34(1):65–8.

[24] Lopez AM, Williams PL, Ampel NM. Acute pulmonary coccidioidomycosis mimicking bacterial pneumonia and septic shock: a report of two cases. Am J Med 1993;95(2): 236–9.

[25] Muntz FH. Oxalate-producing pulmonary aspergillosis in an alpaca. Vet Pathol 1999;36(6):631–2.

[26] Grooters AM. Pythiosis, lagenidiosis, and zygomycosis in small animals. Vet Clin North Am Small Anim Pract 2003;33(4):695–720.

[27] Legendre AM, Becker PU. Evaluation of the agar-gel immunodiffusion test in the diagnosis of canine blastomycosis. Am J Vet Res 1980;41(12):2109–11.

[28] Greene CE, editor. Histoplasmosis. In: Infectious diseases of the dog and cat. 3rd edition. St. Louis (MO): Sauders Elseiver; 2006. p. 378–83.

[29] Flatland B, Greene RT, Lappin MR. Clinical and serologic evaluation of cats with cryptococcosis. J Am Vet Med Assoc 1996;209(6):1110–3.

[30] Tang Y-W, Li H, Durkin MM, et al. Urine polymerase chain reaction is not as sensitive as urine antigen for the diagnosis of disseminated histoplasmosis. Diagn Microbiol Infect Dis 2006;54(4):283–7.

[31] Marr KA, Balajee SA, McLaughlin L, et al. Detection of galactomannan antigenemia by enzyme immunoassay for the diagnosis of invasive aspergillosis: variables that affect performance. J Infect Dis 2004;190(3):641–9.

[32] Shurley JF, Legendre AM, Scalarone GM. Blastomyces dermatitidis antigen detection in urine specimens from dogs with blastomycosis using a competitive binding inhibition ELISA. Mycopathologia 2005;160(2):137–42.

[33] Wheat J, Wheat H, Connolly P, et al. Cross-reactivity in Histoplasma capsulatum variety capsulatum antigen assays of urine samples from patients with endemic mycoses. Clin Infect Dis 1997;24(6):1169–71.

[34] Grooters AM, Leise BS, Lopez MK, et al. Development and evaluation of an enzyme-linked immunosorbent assay for the serodiagnosis of pythiosis in dogs. J Vet Intern Med 2002; 16(2):142–6.

[35] Shubitz LE, Butkiewicz CD, Dial SM, et al. Incidence of coccidioides infection among dogs residing in a region in which the organism is endemic. J Am Vet Med Assoc 2005;226(11): 1846–50.

[36] Ampel NM. Emerging disease issues and fungal pathogens associated with HIV infection. Emerg Infect Dis 1996;2(2):109–16.

[37] Wheat JL. Current diagnosis of histoplasmosis. Trends Microbiol 2003;11(10):488–94.

[38] Newman SJ, Langston CE, Scase TJ. Cryptococcal pyelonephritis in a dog. J Am Vet Med Assoc 2003;222(2):180–3.

[39] Grooters AM, Gee MK. Development of a nested polymerase chain reaction assay for the detection and identification of Pythium insidiosum. J Vet Intern Med 2002;16(2): 147–52.

[40] Gene J, Blanco JL, Cano J, et al. New filamentous fungus Sagenomella chlamydospora responsible for a disseminated infection in a dog. J Clin Microbiol 2003;41(4):1722–5.

[41] Abramo F, Vercelli A, Mancianti F. Two cases of dermatophytic pseudomycetoma in the dog: an immunohistochemical study. Vet Dermatol 2001;12:203–7.

[42] Brown CC, McClure JJ, Triche P, et al. Use of immunohistochemical methods for diagnosis of equine pythiosis. Am J Vet Res 1988;49(11):1866–8.

[43] Patton CS, Hake R, Newton J, et al. Esophagitis due to Pythium insidiosum infection in two dogs. J Vet Intern Med 1996;10(3):139–42.

[44] Byrd J, Mehregan DR, Mehregan DA. Utility of anti-bacillus Calmette-Guerin antibodies as a screen for organisms in sporotrichoid infections. J Am Acad Dermatol 2001;44(2): 261–4.

[45] Bonenberger TE, Ihrke PJ, Naydan DK, et al. Rapid identification of tissue micro-organisms in skin biopsy specimens from domestic animals using polyclonal BCG antibody. Vet Dermatol 2001;12(1):41–7.

[46] Available at: http://ihc.sdstate.org.

[47] Available at: http://pcr.sdstate.org.

[48] Atkins SD, Clark IM. Fungal molecular diagnostics: a mini review. J Appl Genet 2004; 45(1):3–15.

[49] Malorny B, Tassios PT, Radstrom P, et al. Standardization of diagnostic PCR for the detection of foodborne pathogens. Int J Food Microbiol 2003;83(1):39–48.

[50] Wallace PS. Linkage between the journal and Quality Control Molecular Diagnostics (QCMD). J Clin Virol 2003;27(3):211–2.

[51] Tichopad A, Didier A, Pfaffl MW. Inhibition of real-time RT-PCR quantification due to tissue-specific contaminants. Mol Cell Probes 2004;18(1):45–50.

[52] Garcia ME, Duran C, Cruzado M, et al. Evaluation of molecular and immunological techniques for the diagnosis of mammary aspergillosis in ewes. Vet Microbiol 2004;98(1): 17–21.

[53] Kano R, Fujino Y, Takamoto N, et al. PCR detection of the Cryptococcus neoformans CAP59 gene from a biopsy specimen from a case of feline cryptococcosis. J Vet Diagn Invest 2001;13:439–42.

[54] Znajda NR, Grooters AM, Marsella R. PCR-based detection of Pythium and Lagenidium DNA in frozen and ethanol-fixed animal tissues. Vet Dermatol 2002;13:187–94.

[55] Ueda Y, Sano A, Tamura M, et al. Diagnosis of histoplasmosis by detection of internal transcribed spacer region of fungal rRNA gene from a paraffin-embedded skin sample from a dog in Japan. Vet Microbiol 2003;94:219–24.

[56] Millar BC, Jiru X, Walker MJ, et al. False identification of Coccidioides immitis: do molecular methods always get it right? J Clin Microbiol 2003;41(12):5778–80.

[57] Cai HY, Archambault M, Gyles CL, et al. Molecular genetic methods in the veterinary clinical bacteriology laboratory: current usage and future applications. Anim Health Res Rev 2003;4(2):73–93.

[58] Nordstrom H, Johansson P, Li QG, et al. Microarray technology for identification and distinction of hantaviruses. J Med Virol 2004;72(4):646–55.

[59] Rementeria A, Lopez-Molina N, Ludwig A, et al. Genes and molecules involved in Aspergillus fumigatus virulence. Rev Iberoam Micol 2005;22(1):1–23.

[60] Felipe MS, Andrade RV, Arraes FB, et al. Transcriptional profiles of the human pathogenic fungus Paracoccidioides brasiliensis in mycelium and yeast cells. J Biol Chem 2005; 280(26):24706–14.

Vet Clin Small Anim 37 (2007) 393–402

VETERINARY CLINICS
SMALL ANIMAL PRACTICE

Getting the Most from Dermatopathology

Gregory A. Campbell, MS, DVM, PhD[a],*,
Leslie Sauber, DVM[b]

[a]Oklahoma Animal Disease Diagnostic Laboratory, Oklahoma State
University Center for Veterinary Health Sciences, Farm Road and Ridge Road,
Stillwater, OK 74078, USA
[b]Tulsa Veterinary Dermatology, 7220 East 41st Street, Tulsa, OK 74145, USA

D ermatologic diseases are common sources of frustration for clients and veterinarians alike. The most frustrating situations often arise when a definitive diagnosis has not been made or when secondary problems like pyoderma complicate or obscure the primary dermatologic problem. Many frequently used diagnostic tests are inexpensive and are technically easy to perform and interpret. These include skin scrapings, dermatophyte cultures, cutaneous cytology, and trichograms. Veterinarians perform these tests routinely and are confident in their procurement of samples and in the interpretation of their findings. These tests often lead to a definitive diagnosis or are used to rule out specific diagnoses.

Dermatohistopathology is one of the most powerful diagnostic tools in clinical dermatology. It is a process in which the veterinary clinician and the veterinary pathologist must consider themselves a team in patient care.

The veterinary clinician must:

1. Know when biopsies are indicated
2. Be able to select lesions to biopsy that are likely to yield diagnostic results
3. Skillfully procure the biopsy samples
4. Provide the pathologist with an accurate history, clinical description, and clinical differential diagnosis

The pathologist must:

1. Have particular interest and expertise in dermatohistopathology
2. Be readily accessible to the clinician
3. Be vigilant in the pursuit of an accurate histologic description and interpretation

In attention to these detailed steps in the process can lead to nonspecific, nondiagnostic, or even misleading results. Dermatohistopathology can thus also be

*Corresponding author. E-mail address: gregory.campbell@okstate.edu (G.A. Campbell).

0195-5616/07/$ – see front matter
doi:10.1016/j.cvsm.2006.11.007

an added source of frustration for the clinician. In the following discussion, the authors discuss the clinician's and pathologist's roles in getting the most out of dermatohistopathology.

CLINICIAN'S ROLE IN DERMATOHISTOPATHOLOGY

Selection of Cases

Dermatohistopathology can serve in the diagnosis of many different types of skin diseases. Indications for skin biopsies are therefore numerous and rules for when to perform a biopsy are not absolute. The following are guidelines that the authors have found to be helpful:

1. All cases of suspected neoplasia: excisional biopsies are indicated if the excision of a single or a few tumors could be curative. Incisional biopsies should be performed when there are multiple or large tumors or when therapies other than excision are likely to be indicated (eg, suspected cutaneous lymphoma, large infiltrative tumors on extremities in which amputation may be indicated).

2. When dermatologic signs are not responding to rational therapy: for example, most canine pustules are caused by superficial pyoderma with *Staphylococcus intermedius* organisms. If a patient with pustules and epidermal collarettes is not responding to traditionally effective antistaphylococcal treatments, biopsies should be performed to rule out other causes of superficial pustules, such as pemphigus foliaceus or subcorneal pustular dermatosis. Similarly, dogs with hypothyroidism that have not responded to adequate thyroxine supplementation should have biopsies to rule out other causes of nonpruritic alopecia and scaling, such as sebaceous adenitis, follicular dysplasia, or primary keratinization defects.

3. When dermatologic signs are suspected to be associated with internal disease: dermatohistopathologic findings may then guide the veterinarian to pursue additional appropriate diagnostic testing. For example, dermatohistopathologic findings suggestive of hepatocutaneous syndrome would prompt the clinician to evaluate liver function. Findings suggestive of nodular dermatofibrosis would prompt ultrasound evaluation for renal cysts, cystadenomas, and uterine leiomyomas.

4. Chronic ulcerative lesions: such lesions can result from neoplasia, actinic keratosis, or resistant or unusual infectious agents that may require histopathology for a definitive diagnosis.

5. When a suspected disease would require therapy that has serious potential side effects, is expensive, or is time-consuming: examples include autoimmune diseases that require immunosuppression with potentially toxic drugs and primary keratinization disorders that require expensive systemic retinoid therapy and frequent labor-intensive topical shampoo therapy.

6. When dermatohistopathology is the only definitive way to diagnose the suspected disease: many disparate dermatologic diseases fall into this category; examples include follicular dysplasia, autoimmune diseases, and sebaceous adenitis.

7. When specific infectious diseases are suspected: certain infectious agents, such as mycobacterial organisms, are difficult to culture or may be slow to

grow in the microbiology laboratory. Demonstration of organisms on dermatohistopathology may yield a much more rapid and accurate diagnosis than culture alone. Certain fungal disease, such as the systemic mycoses (eg, blastomycosis, coccidioidomycosis, histoplasmosis), are potentially infectious to microbiology laboratory personnel. Formalin-fixed tissues are not infectious; thus, they provide a diagnosis while keeping laboratory workers safe. In these cases, dermatohistopathology may be preferred to microbial culturing.

8. When lesions are unusual or develop in unusual sites: even experienced veterinarians only encounter rare skin diseases on rare occasions. Therefore, they may not readily recognize clinical signs associated with conditions like hepatocutaneous syndrome, nevi, or Vogt-Kayanagi-Harada–like syndrome.

It is also important to recognize when biopsies are unlikely to be diagnostically useful and are therefore not indicated. The most common examples are chronic pruritic allergic dermatitis or parasitic dermatitis. Dermatohistopathology of these diseases is often nonspecific: "epidermal hyperplasia and mixed perivascular inflammation consistent with allergic or parasitic skin disease" is a typical finding that does not add to the clinician's understanding of the disease process. The diagnosis of allergic disease is made on the basis of historical findings, clinical signs, and ruling out other pruritic diseases. The diagnosis of parasitic disease is made on the basis of skin scrapings or treatment trials with appropriate antiparasiticidal therapy.

Finally, it should be stressed that dermatohistopathology is not a substitute for clinical acumen. Submitting samples before collecting an accurate history, performing a detailed physical examination, and formulating differential diagnoses often results in histologic findings that are not clinically useful.

Timing of the Biopsy Procedure

Dermatohistopathology is most diagnostic when samples are taken early in the disease process while pristine primary lesions are present. Many dermatologic diseases quickly become secondarily infected with commensal organisms, however. This is a particularly common problem in dogs, which readily develop secondary superficial pyoderma, bacterial folliculitis, and *Malassezia* dermatitis. These secondary infections often obscure the clinical and histologic pictures. If lesions are secondarily infected, it behooves the clinician to treat the infection first and to postpone the biopsy procedure until the secondary infections have resolved.

Lesion Selection

Once the clinician has decided to perform skin biopsies, lesion selection is the next critical step. Dermatologic diseases often present with a variety of gross lesions that may appear simultaneously or in progression over time. Evaluation of different lesion types and lesions from various body sites yields the most complete histologic picture. Multiple samples are therefore almost always indicated. Gross lesions are characterized as primary or secondary in nature. Primary lesions are diagnostically much more significant than secondary lesions and should be sampled when present. It is therefore essential that the clinician have a thorough understanding of primary and secondary skin lesions.

Primary skin lesions are the initial eruptions that develop spontaneously as a direct reflection of the underlying disease. These lesions appear early in the course of the disease but may quickly become obscured by secondary lesions. Primary lesions include macules, patches, papules, plaques, pustules, vesicles, bullae, wheals, nodules, tumors, and cysts [1]. Accurate identification of gross primary lesions often leads the clinician to a relatively limited clinical differential diagnosis. For example, relatively few disease processes result in pustules. The most common include superficial pyoderma, pemphigus foliaceus, and subcorneal pustular dermatosis. Identification of these gross lesions therefore significantly limits the differential diagnosis for the clinician. In much the same way, histopathology of primary lesions often leads the pathologist to a definitive or limited differential diagnosis. Furthermore, the pathologist can often distinguish between pustules caused by superficial pyoderma and those caused by pemphigus foliaceus. Therefore, when primary lesions are present, they should always be sampled.

Secondary lesions evolve from primary lesions or are a result of self-trauma or topical or systemic medications. Secondary lesions include epidermal collarettes, scars, excoriations, erosions, ulcers, fissures, lichenification, and calluses [1]. These lesions are less specific than primary lesions; however, in some cases, they may still provide gross clues for the clinician. For example, epidermal collarettes are suggestive of previous pustules, vesicles, or bulla. This would result in a clinical differential diagnosis that includes the causes of these primary lesions. Other secondary lesions are more nonspecific. For example, lichenification and hyperpigmentation commonly occur with chronic dermatosis from a disparate group of diseases, and thus are not helpful in formulating a clinical differential diagnosis.

In the same manner, histopathologic findings of secondary lesions are also frequently nonspecific. In the case of an epidermal collarette, the pathologist would not typically be able to differentiate whether the collarette had been caused by a pustule versus a vesicle. In the case of lichenification and hyperpigmentation, the pathologist would note that these changes are attributable to chronic dermatosis; although this is significant clinically, it is not new information for the clinician, owner, or pet. Therefore, when secondary lesions alone are sampled, results are often nonspecific and become a source of frustration for the clinician and the pathologist.

Still other gross lesions can be primary or secondary depending on the pathogenesis of the condition. These include alopecia, scale, crusts, follicular casts, comedones, hyperpigmentation, and hypopigmentation [1]. When the lesion is suspected as primary, biopsies of that lesion are indicated. If the lesion is secondary, biopsy findings are likely to be nonspecific. For example, hair shaft breakage associated with follicular dysplasia leads to primary alopecia, whereas pruritic allergic dermatitis leads to self-trauma and subsequent secondary alopecia. Histopathology is not only indicated when follicular dysplasia is suspected but is the only method to diagnose this disease definitively. Conversely, histopathology of secondary alopecia attributable to allergic skin disease is usually nonspecific and does not provide any new information to the clinician.

Finally, if lesions appear on different areas of the body, samples from each area should be taken. Examples include vesicles or pustules appearing on mucous membranes and skin and hyperkeratosis or scaling of haired skin and foot pads.

Biopsy Techniques

Biopsies are performed using a biopsy punch or excision with a scalpel. Punch biopsies are most commonly performed because they are technically simple; quick to perform; and provide samples of the epidermis, dermis, and superficial subcutis that are adequate for the diagnosis of most dermatologic diseases. A 6-mm punch is the standard size used because this usually provides a large enough sample size yet is small enough to be easily blocked with local anesthesia. A 4-mm punch may be necessary for more delicate areas, such as the nasal planum, eyelids, pinnae, and foot pads.

The selected biopsy site should not be surgically prepared because this can remove skin surface lesions. Light clipping of hair on and surrounding the biopsy site may be necessary to facilitate visualization, however. Local anesthesia, such as infiltration of the subcutis with 1% to 2% lidocaine, is usually adequate for truncal lesions. General anesthesia is usually necessary for biopsies of the face, nasal planum, pinnae, and feet or when larger samples are taken with a scalpel.

When using a biopsy punch, the instrument should be centered directly over the lesion and should not include any significant amount of normal skin (see section on trimming of samples). The punch is ideally aligned along the direction of the hair shaft. To minimize artifacts arising from shearing forces, the punch should be rotated in only one direction. Once the punch has penetrated into the subcutis, the instrument is carefully withdrawn. Nontraumatic forceps should be used to grasp the sample gently at its attachment to the subcutis, thus avoiding crushing of the epidermis and dermis with surgical instruments. The attachment is then cut from the subcutis with small curved scissors.

When larger or deeper biopsies are indicated, punch biopsies may be inadequate, making it necessary to obtain biopsies using a scalpel. Specific examples include resectable tumors and lesions that involve the deep subcutis. Delicate primary lesions, such as vesicles, bullae, or pustules, may rupture during the shearing motion of a punch biopsy and may be best obtained with a scalpel.

Once the sample has been excised, it should be gently blotted to remove excessive blood and immediately placed in a formalin vial. Biopsies taken from areas of the skin with a thin dermis (eg, pinna, ventral abdomen) or long linear samples may curl and become distorted when fixed in formalin. This makes it difficult for the histopathology laboratory to orient the samples properly for sectioning. To avoid this, samples can be blotted and then placed subcutis side down onto a small substrate, such as a piece of cardboard or wooden tongue depressor, for 1 to 2 minutes. Once the sample is slightly adhered to the substrate, the entire sample (substrate with attached biopsy specimen) should be placed into the formalin vial.

After the biopsy has been performed, the surgical site can be clipped and scrubbed before closing with skin sutures. This results in a more cosmetic postoperative biopsy site for the owner.

Provide an Accurate Clinical Picture to the Pathologist

The clinician uses the signalment, history, and clinical findings to produce a clinical differential diagnosis. The pathologist uses dermatohistopathologic findings to produce a histologic differential diagnosis. When these tools are combined, the differential can often be narrowed or prioritized. The clinician must therefore provide the pathologist with detailed clinical information.

The signalment may alert the clinician and pathologist to specific breed-, gender-, or age-related diseases. For example, comedones are considered normal findings for alopecic breeds, such Chinese Crested dogs or Sphinx cats, and may not be diagnostically significant. Sertoli cell tumor would need to be included in the differential diagnosis of an intact male dog but not in that of female dogs or neutered male dogs with histologic findings suggestive of "endocrine dermatosis." Age can also be a diagnostic clue. Sterile pyogranulomatous dermatitis in dogs can have many causes, but if the patient is less than 4 months of age, canine juvenile cellulitis would be high on the differential diagnosis list.

Pertinent historical facts include age of onset, progression of signs, and response to medications. Knowledge of a positive or negative response to specific medications is obviously diagnostically significant to the clinician. These findings can also be helpful to the pathologist. Treatment details should be provided in a manner that is meaningful to the pathologist. For example, reporting that a patient with pustular dermatosis "did not respond to cefpodoxime proxetil therapy" may not be meaningful to a pathologist who is not familiar with the treatment of pyoderma or the drug cefpodoxime proxetil. Reporting that this same patient "did not respond to antibiotics that are traditionally effective for superficial pyoderma" may be much more useful to the pathologist.

Physical examination findings, especially identification of lesion types, is not only important when formulating a clinical differential and in biopsy site selection as discussed previously but is also important information to provide to the pathologist. If the clinician reports that pustules are present and has submitted appropriate samples, the pathologist should specifically look for the pustules in the processed samples. If they are not present, the pathologist can request recuts or request that the clinician provide additional biopsies from pustules.

Distribution of the lesions can also be revealing. For example, discoid lupus erythematosus is most commonly confined to the skin of the face, whereas other types of autoimmune disease, such as pemphigus foliaceus, usually present with more generalized lesions. Furthermore, because the histology of normal skin varies between anatomic sites, it is imperative that the pathologist receive specific information regarding the anatomic location from which a biopsy was taken. Only then is the pathologist able to interpret the microscopic findings accurately. For example, normal epidermis of the nasal planum and foot pads is extremely thick compared with haired skin. Criteria for epidermal hyperplasia or hypoplasia are significantly different between these sites.

Finally, the clinician should provide a working clinical differential diagnosis that acts to open a dialog between the clinician and the pathologist. The clinician is asking, "I suspect this specific disease, group of diseases, or general disease process. Can you help me determine which, if any, of these diseases are most likely?" The pathologist answers by specifically addressing the differential list and by adding any additional differentials that are suggested by dermatohistopathology.

The dialog should continue if the clinician does not think that the histologic diagnosis correlates with the clinical picture. The pathologist should be directly consulted, and the case should be discussed in more detail. This discussion may prompt the pathologist to re-evaluate the slides, order new sections from the histology laboratory, or recommend special stains or immunohistochemistry. The discussion may also prompt the clinician to consider other diagnostic tests, such as endocrine testing, cultures, or routine blood work.

Choosing a Dermatohistopathologist

From the previous discussion, it is clear that the ideal pathologist is one with particular interest and expertise in dermatohistopathology. One way of finding such a pathologist is to seek recommendation from the veterinary dermatologist to whom you refer your difficult dermatologic cases. Dermatologists often have a close working relationship with their pathologist and should feel confident in referring you to him or her. At some veterinary colleges, dermatologists and pathologists meet regularly to review and discuss clinical cases and histologic findings. Some groups welcome outside submissions from general practitioners. Contact the various veterinary colleges to find out if one of these groups is right for you.

Once a pathologist is chosen, familiarity and mutual respect are paramount in establishing a good working relationship. This takes time and effort but results in more accurate diagnostic capabilities, which help to attain the ultimate goal of better patient care.

PATHOLOGIST'S ROLE IN DERMATOHISTOPATHOLOGY

The role of the pathologist in any case is to provide accessible, accountable, and vigilant diagnostic services for veterinary clinicians. It would be an ideal world if the pathologist's role in dermatohistopathology was simply to examine sections from a skin biopsy and provide a diagnosis. Because of the relatively limited response of skin to insult or injury, the diagnosis of "chronic hyperplastic perivascular dermatitis" or similar seemingly nonspecific diagnoses without clinical correlation can be frustrating for the pathologist and clinician alike. In an excellent article by Dunstan [2], an overview of the process, beginning with tissue fixation and ending with histologic evaluation, is provided. A summary is provided here with updates on more recent practices.

Tissue Fixation

The most commonly used fixative for skin biopsy specimens is 10% neutral buffered formalin. This is frequently provided by diagnostic laboratories in appropriately labeled shipping containers with appropriate quantities for small specimens. In the past, Michel's fixative was necessary for performing immunofluorescence staining to identify autoantibodies to aid in the diagnosis of immune-mediated skin disease. Today, most laboratories rely on immunohistochemical staining to identify autoantibodies, however. This testing is performed on routine formalin-fixed and paraffin-embedded tissue specimens, thus negating the need to submit additional samples in Michel's fixative. Furthermore, the field of immunohistochemistry is rapidly expanding to include identification of cell markers used in the diagnosis of neoplasms as well as infectious agents in tissue sections.

Trimming, Processing, and Staining of Fixed Tissue

In most diagnostic laboratories, samples are routed to a trimming area, where a technician is responsible for orienting and properly trimming specimens. Most routine punch biopsy specimens are bisected with the two halves submitted for processing and embedding. This usually presents no problems but can induce significant artifact in specific instances. One situation in which this arises is in trimming biopsy specimens from cases with the primary presenting complaint of alopecia. Ideally, punch biopsy specimens are trimmed in the direction of hair growth, resulting in histologic sections that are in the longitudinal plane of hair follicles. When no hair is present on the specimen surface, proper trimming can be problematic. A simple technique at the time of biopsy is to draw a line on the skin surface paralleling the direction of hair growth using a permanent marker. This provides a landmark for trimming the specimen by the laboratory.

A second situation that frequently causes the tissue trimmer problems is when a circular punch is used to perform a biopsy of the margin of a lesion to provide lesional skin and adjacent normal skin. These are difficult to orient properly because most circular punch specimens are simply bisected before processing. If the line of bisection does not occur across the border of the lesion, one can end up with essentially normal skin and a nondiagnostic specimen. It is more appropriate in these cases to provide punch specimens from the lesion and adjacent nonlesional skin.

Nodular lesions or tumors are commonly received as elliptically shaped specimens with the lesion located centrally, or smaller portions of a larger specimen are received. Because of time and cost constraints, evaluation of excisional margins is typically limited. Some diagnostic laboratories have extra charges for more extensive margin evaluation. Commercially available colored dyes (Davidson Marking System; Bradley Products, Bloomington, Minnesota) can be used to paint the margins of a larger specimen at the time of excision and before fixation. These dyes are provided in different colors, and individual colors can be applied to different margins. These are applied to blotted fresh tissue and allowed to remain on the tissue for 2 to 5 minutes before formalin fixation. These remain on the surface of the specimen through processing and can provide a better evaluation of excisional margins in many cases, especially with larger excised masses. An economic means of accomplishing the same goal is to use India ink for painting margins.

Most diagnostic laboratories currently use automated tissue processing, embedding, and staining equipment, resulting in much less frequent induction of artifact in this critical step of tissue handling. With current techniques, turnaround time for routine specimens has been significantly shortened.

The most commonly used routine stain for tissue examination is hematoxylin-eosin. This is generally adequate for evaluation of most specimens. If there are histologic findings, such as deep pyogranulomatous inflammation or periadnexal inflammation, additional stains may be indicated to rule out the presence of organisms. Gomori's methenamine silver (GMS) and periodic acid–Schiff (PAS) are stains commonly used for detection of fungi. Fite's acid-fast stain is used for identification of acid-fast positive bacteria. Some mast cell tumors may not be readily identifiable in routine sections. In those cases, Giemsa or toluidine blue stain can be useful in identifying mast cell granules. Because of the extra labor and expense involved, many diagnostic laboratories charge extra for additional stains. After staining, slides are permanently coverslipped and are ready for examination. A good dermatohistopathologist is familiar with the indications for special stains and should order these stains promptly. A good clinician should also be aware of the indications for special stains, however, and can indicate in the animal's history if stains may be indicated.

In some cases of cutaneous neoplasia, the pathologist may arrive at the histologic diagnosis of "round cell tumor" or "spindle cell tumor" based on routine stains. In many of these cases, immunohistochemical stains can be used to identify the cell type present more specifically. Immunohistochemical staining technique simply involves the use of antibodies directed against specific cell components, which can be internal or cell surface components. The commonly used immunostains can be performed on routine, formalin-fixed, and paraffin-embedded tissues. Tissue sections are incubated with the antibody for the cell marker in question. The binding of the primary antibody to tissue components is detected using a specific secondary antibody, followed by a step that develops a colored reaction product at the site of binding. The same technique can be used to identify viruses, bacteria, and parasites in tissue sections with primary antibodies directed against antigenic components of those organisms. There is typically an extra charge for these stains. Antibodies used can cost upward of $200 to $1000 per milliliter, and it requires technical time and special equipment to perform these special techniques.

Dermatohistopathologic Examination

Histologic examination and generation of a meaningful report is a crucial step in getting the most from dermatopathology. When a pathologist initially examines a biopsy specimen, recognition of stereotypic reactions of the skin and patterns of inflammatory and neoplastic infiltration are the primary initial diagnostic tools used. This "pattern analysis" approach is often sufficient to provide an accurate diagnosis and prognosis with a relatively rapid turnaround time. A few examples of such conditions include atrophic diseases of the epidermis or hair follicles, diseases with abnormal cornification, pustular disease involving the epidermis, bullous diseases, interface lesions, perivascular inflammation, and vasculitis [3]. Each of these histologic patterns, although not always diagnostically specific, usually limits the list of differential diagnoses to rule out.

On completion of the histologic examination, the pathologist correlates the provided history with the clinical diagnosis and usually provides an interpretive comment and prognosis.

Final Analysis

Detailed attention to the procurement of samples by the clinician and evaluation of biopsy samples by the pathologist are obviously necessary for accurate results but do not represent the final step. Once the clinician receives the pathology report, he or she has the arduous task of correlating the clinical findings with the pathologic findings. If the pathologic findings are supportive of the clinical findings, dermatohistopathology is immediately rewarding. If the pathologic findings do not fit the clinical picture, a dialog with the pathologist should be opened. A good pathologist appreciates interaction with the clinician as part of the team whose goal it is to provide an accurate diagnosis that leads to the best patient care.

References

[1] Scott DW, Miller WH, Griffin CE. Muller and Kirk's small animal dermatology. 6th edition. Philadelphia: WB Saunders; 2000. p. 86–7.
[2] Dunstan RW. A user's guide to veterinary surgical pathology laboratories. Vet Clin North Am Small Anim Pract 1990;20(6):1397–417.
[3] Yager JA, Wilcock BP. Color atlas and text of surgical pathology of the dog and cat; dermatopathology and skin tumors. London: Mosby-Year Book Europe Limited; 1994. p. 15–41.

INDEX

Note: Page numbers of article titles are in **boldface** type.

0195-5616/07/$ – see front matter
doi:10.1016/S0195-5616(07)00020-4

Moving?

Make sure your subscription moves with you!

To notify us of your new address, find your **Clinics Account Number** (located on your mailing label above your name), and contact customer service at:

E-mail: elspcs@elsevier.com

800-654-2452 (subscribers in the U.S. & Canada)
407-345-4000 (subscribers outside of the U.S. & Canada)

Fax number: 407-363-9661

Elsevier Periodicals Customer Service
6277 Sea Harbor Drive
Orlando, FL 32887-4800

*To ensure uninterrupted delivery of your subscription, please notify us at least 4 weeks in advance of move.